A Handbook on Veterinary Local Anaesthesia

Syed Sajjad Hussain
M.V.Sc., Ph.D., FNAVS
Formerly Professor & Head
Division of Surgery & Radiology
& Dean, Faculty of Veterinary Sciences & Animal Husbandry
SKUAST-K, Shuhama, Shalimar, Sri Nagar, J & K
Presently Project Planning & Monitoring Officer
SKUAST-K, Shalimar, Sri Nagar - 191 121, J & K.

International Book Distributing Co.
(Publishing Division)

Published by
International Book Distributing Co.

(Publishing Division)
Chaman Studio Building, 2nd Floor,
Charbagh, Lucknow 226 004 U.P. (INDIA)
Tel. : Off. : 2450004, 2450007, 2459058 Fax : 0522-2458629
E-Mail : ibdco@sancharnet.in

First Edition 2006

Price:

ISBN 81-8189-158-9

Composed & Designed at :
Panacea Computers
3rd Floor, Agrawal Sabha Bhawan
Subhash Mohal, Sadar Cantt. Lucknow-226 002
Phone : 0522-2483312, 9335927082
E-mail : prasgupt@rediffmail.com

Printed at:
Salasar Imaging Systems
C-7/5, Lawrence Road Industrial Area
Delhi - 110 035
Tel. : 011-27185653, 9810064311

Dedicated

To My

Beloved Parents

Ama and Abaji

Who are physically no more with me but continue to inspire me through their unending love and affection and to ARU's for being with me

Prof. Anwar Alam
Vice-Chancellor

S.K. University of Agricultural Science and Technology of Kashmir
Shalimar, Srinagar - 191 121

Foreword

The illustrated Hand Book on "Veterinary Local Anaesthesia" authored by Dr. Syed Sajjad Hussain, Professor-cum-Chief Scientist, Veterinary Surgery & Radiology, former Dean, Faculty of Veterinary Sciences & Animal Husbandry, presently Project Planning and Monitoring Officer, SKUAST-K Shalimar is certainly a contribution towards veterinary science particularly veterinary surgery. It will definitely prove a very useful reference book for the field veterinarians - academicians - students of the stream.

The book gives details of different techniques elucidated by the author through varied techniques evolved and adopted by him while carrying out research on the subject experimented on the experimental animals duly supported by comprehensive illustrations. Local anaesthetic techniques are often required under field conditions by veterinarians, as sophisticated and costly equipments for general anaesthesia are not affordable. I have a considered opinion that the book shall be more useful for practicing veterinarians.

I compliment Dr. Syed Sajjad Hussain, for his work and its comprehensive transformation into a well authored book.

(Prof. Anwar Alam)

Preface

In the world of science there has been a knowledge explosion with evolution of new horizons every moment. The unraveling of newer facts of chemical and biological spheres is leading from specialization to super-specialization making it not only difficult but impossible for any one to keep track of everything. Developments in the field of anaesthesiology viz-a-viz anaesthetics and anaesthetic techniques, is no exception. Anaesthesiology is an important applied science seminal to any surgical intervention. A practicing veterinarian is faced with many problems-

1. He has to deal with varied animal species
2. Non-availability of any specialized anaesthesiologist.
3. Under field circumstances a veterinarian usually finds it difficult to arrange a sophisticated apparatus and general anaesthetic drugs
4. Use of general anaesthesia is economically not viable.
5. The general anaesthetic drugs are contra-indicated in bovines especially under field conditions.

Moreover, in the field it is the Veterinary Assistant Surgeon/ Veterinary Graduate rather than a specialist surgeon who is to undertake the emergency surgical intervention under local and regional anaesthesia. Hence a need was felt to capsulate the vast knowledge to provide the students and practicing veterinarians the important information in an applied fashion and at the same time keeping track of the latest developments in the field. It is the first time an attempt has been made to compile a book on regional and local anaesthesia being practiced in animals. The book includes information on anaesthetic drugs and techniques commonly used in regional and local anaesthesia. A detailed description of different techniques being practiced in different animals especially bovines have been provided along with illustrations depicting the common techniques being performed in animals. In an effort to provide space for new techniques, the intra peritoneal visceral procaine block and long-acting epidural anaesthetic technique has been outlined. The purpose of this handbook is to provide complete and concise information about regional and local anaesthetic techniques being used for all types of operations especially in bovines. We hope the handbook shall provide the necessary technical know-how to overcome any surgical maneuver.

Prof. Syed Sajjad Hussain

Acknowledgements

The author desires to acknowledge the moral support, and the dedicated efforts of many individuals who have helped in bringing out this treatise. Some of them deserve a special mention:

Dr. B.A. Moulvi, Associate Professor-cum-Senior Scientist, Veterinary Surgery and Radiology, was not only involved in conception of this endeavour but also kept a track of the manuscript, suggesting improvements at every point. The author has found his suggestions a distillation of his experiences in teaching the professional graduates and post-graduates.

Dr. Mudasir Sultana, Assistant Professor, Veterinary Pharmacology, painstakingly went through the manuscript. Her suggestions have been duly incorporated and thankfully acknowledged.

Dr. J.D. Parrah, Assistant Professor, Veterinary Surgery and Radiology, put a final polish to the manuscript, combined text and figures, and eliminated stylistic and typographical errors.

Dr. M.S. Mir, Assistant Professor, Veterinary Pathology designed the textbook's typography and its covers.

Mr. Nazar-ul-Islam, helped in typesetting of the manuscript.

The author feels indebted to **Dr. Amresh Kumar**, Dean, College of Veterinary Sciences and Animal Husbandry, GB Pant Agricultural University for his valuable suggestions.

Prof. Syed Sajjad Hussain
Prof. & Head
Division of Surgery & Radiology,
Dean, Faculty of Veterinary Sciences
& Animal Husbandry
SKUAST-K, Shuhama

Contents

1.	Introduction	1
2.	Common Terminology	3
3.	Central and Peripheral Nervous System	7
4.	Anatomy and Physiology of Peripheral Nerves	10
5.	Local Anaesthetics	16
6.	Pharmacological Properties and Mechanism of Action of Local Analgesics	20
7.	Clinically Common Local Analgesics	24
8.	Local Analgesic Techniques	28
9.	Therapeutic Local Anaesthetic Blocks	34
10.	Regional Analgesia	50
11.	Regional Anaesthesia Techniques	57
12.	Regional Anaesthetic Blocks of the Fore Limb	69
13.	Nerve Blocks of Hind Limb	79
14.	Use of Preanaesthetics in Animals	94
15.	Neurolept Analgesics	106
16.	Systemic and Toxic Effects of Local Analgesics	109
17.	Acupuncture Anaesthesia	112
	Index	118

1 Introduction

Local analgesia denotes transitory loss of sensibility in a defined part of the body. It is caused by direct delivery of local anaesthetic to peripheral neural targets with the primary goal of interrupting conduction of afferent nerve impulse. Regional anaesthesia signifies insensibility induced by blocking the major nerves of the given region without piercing the region itself. The anaesthetic agents obtund sensation and reduce motor tone in the innervated areas distal to the site of application without depressing consciousness or sensation in the other parts of the body. The local and regional anaesthetic blocks are employed to perform different surgical operations in animals. Many surgical operations in standing animals are most desirable and are very conveniently performed under these blocks. The local analgesics are the drugs that produce reversible neural blockade by impeding impulse transmission in perineural nerves, spinal roots, nerve endings, when delivered directly in their vicinity. The use of sedatives before administration of local anaesthetic agents usually is indicated for restraint and management of animals. However, sedatives are avoided when surgical procedures are desired in standing large animals. The local and regional anaesthetic blocks are no more second rate procedures, as these techniques were considered when general anaesthesia was not available. These blocks are commonly viable, as the local anaesthetic agents are less expensive and their application is less time-consuming and requires a few personnel. The techniques of local analgesia are not difficult to learn and their applications do not involve the use of sophisticated or expensive equipments. The purpose of local analgesia in veterinary practice, apart from performance of painless surgery, is also to diagnose lameness in animals. Moreover, it is also being used for therapeutic reasons.

Recent development in local anaesthetic technique, like intraperitoneal visceral blockade, has enabled the veterinary surgeon to induce visceral anaesthesia for abdominal surgery as well as for therapeutic reasons for many ailments in animals. The long-acting epidural anaesthetic techniques have facilitated the performing of protracted surgical maneuvers and provided relief in some chronic cases of ailments in animals.

2 Common Terminology

Acupuncture: A medical treatment from China that involves putting special needles (long and fine) into particular parts of the body to induce analgesia.

Anaesthesia: The word anaesthesia is derived from the Greek for "insensible" or "without feeling". It is used to describe the loss of sensation to the entire or any part of the body. The basic goal of anaesthesia is to create a reversible condition of comfort, quiescence, and physiological stability in a patient before, during, and after performance of a procedure that would otherwise be painful, frightening or hazardous.

Anaesthesiologist: A physician specialist in anesthesiology (in distinction to an anaesthetist who may not be a physician).

Anaesthetist: One who produces anaesthesia by the administration of an anaesthetic drug.

Analeptic (Respiratory): Refers to drugs that stimulate a depressed respiratory centre to produce increased respiratory exchange. In addition to restoring respiratory function, analeptics may restore depressed vasomotor and cerebral functions including consciousness.

Analgesia: Refers to freedom from or absence of pain.

Analgesics: Drugs that cause a temporary loss of the sense of pain without a loss of consciousness. Some act upon the brain or the whole nervous system and are called **anodynes,** while others act locally and are called **local analgesics.**

Anesthesiology: Is defined as the art and science of administration of anaesthesia.

Anaesthetic: A drug that produces anaesthesia.

Ataractic: Is a term used to describe drugs which induce peace of mind. It is a synonymous with tranquilizer.

Axolemma: The plasma membrane bonding the axon is called the axolemma.

Axon: Is the name given to the longest process of cell body. It arises from a small conical elevation on the cell body, devoid of Nissl's granules called **axon hillock**.

Axoplasm: The cytoplasm of the axon is termed the axoplasm.

Basal narcosis: A state of unconsciousness produced by drugs before anaesthesia or operation.

Catalepsy: Is a term applied to a nervous affection characterized by the sudden suspension of sensation and volition, accompanied by a peculiar rigidity of the whole or part of a certain muscle of the body.

Caudal epidural analgesia: Epidural analgesia induced by the injection of a local anaesthetic solution through spaces between the arches of the first and second coccygeal vertebrae into the caudal epidural space.

Conduction anaesthesia: Induced by interruption of nerve conduction by the injection of local analgesic drugs, in proximity to a nerve(s).

Continuous caudal analgesia: Fractional caudal analgesia; a malleable caudal needle or catheter is inserted into the caudal canal and left *in situ* to permit serial intermittent injections of the local analgesic drug for prolonged caudal analgesia.

Continuous spinal analgesia: Fractional caudal analgesia; a malleable spinal needle or catheter is inserted into the spinal subarachnoid space and left *in situ* to permit serial intermittent injections of the local analgesic drug for prolonged spinal analgesia.

Dissociation anaesthesia: Is induced by drugs (e.g., ketamine) that dissociate the thalamocortic and limbic systems. This form of anaesthesia is characterized by a cataleptoid state in which the eyes remain open and swallowing reflexes remain functional.

Electric analgesia: Local analgesia produced by low intensity high frequency electric stimulation of the skin through surface electrodes.

Epidural analgesia: Produced by deposition of local analgesic solution into the epidural space.

Field block analgesia: It is a kind of regional analgesia produced by creating a wall of analgesia around the operative field by the injection of a local analgesic drug.

Hypnosis: Is a condition of artificially induced sleep, or a trance resembling sleep, resulting from moderate depression of CNS from which the patient is readily aroused. This type of CNS alteration is rarely achieved in veterinary patients.

Infiltration analgesia: Induced by the injection of local analgesic solution directly into the tissues that are to be anaesthetized.

Intraosseous analgesia: It is induced by injection of local drugs into bone marrow.

Intravenous local or regional analgesia: A method of producing analgesia in a limb by intravenous injection of local analgesic solution after the limb has been rendered ischaemic by constriction of blood supply with the help of a tourniquet.

Local analgesia: The nerve conduction is blocked and painful impulses fail to reach the brain, when local analgesic drugs are applied locally to nerve tissue in effective concentrations. It is limited to local area.

Narcosis: Is a drug induced deep sleep from which the patient cannot easily be aroused. Narcosis may or may not be accompanied by analgesia.

Neuroglia: The neurons of central nervous system are supported by several varieties of non-excitable cells, which together are called neuroglia.

Paravertebral analgesia: Produced by the injection of local analgesic solution near nerve(s) at its/their exit from the vertebral canal.

Pressure analgesia: Compression analgesia, analgesia induced by pressure applied to a nerve(s).

Refrigeration analgesia: Local analgesia produced by the application of cold with a spray of ethyl chloride or other volatile substances.

Regional analgesia: Produced by injection of local analgesic drug into the connective tissue around a sensory nerve trunk to induce nerve block or field block.

Sedative: The production of state of lessened functional activity of the central nervous system in which the patient is awake but calm.

Segmental analgesia: Loss of sensation limited to an area supplied by one or more spinal nerve roots.

Spinal analgesia: Produced by the injection of an analgesic drug into the spinal subarachnoid space.

Surgical anaesthesia: Inability to feel pain when subjected to surgical stimuli.

Topical or surface analgesia: It results in loss of sensation of the skin or mucous membrane, when the drug is applied to cause loss of sensation by paralyzing the sensory nerve endings.

Tranquilization: State of relaxation and decreased awareness.

3 Central and Peripheral Nervous System

The nervous system is divided into two main parts. The central nervous system which consists of brain and spinal cord, and the peripheral nervous system which consists of cranial and spinal nerves and their associated ganglia. Both brain and spinal cord are covered with membranes, the meninges, and suspended in cerebrospinal fluid. They are further protected by the bone of skull and vertebral column.

The central nervous system is composed of large number of excitable nerve cells and their processes called neurons, which are supported by specialized tissue called neuroglia. The long processes of nerve cells are called axons or nerve fibers. The interior of the central nervous system is organized into gray and white matter. The brain and spinal cord are the main centers where correlation and integration of nervous information occurs.

In the peripheral nervous system, the cranial and spinal nerves, which consist of bundles of nerve fibers or axons conduct information to and from the central nervous system.

Autonomic nervous system

The autonomic nervous system is the part of nervous system concerned with the innervation of involuntary structures such as heart, smooth muscles, and glands within the body. It is distributed throughout the central and peripheral nervous system. The autonomic nervous system may be divided into sympathetic and parasympathetic. The activities of the sympathetic system prepare the body for an emergency whereas the activities of parasympathetic contribute towards conserving and restoring energy.

Major division of the central nervous system

Spinal cord and brain

Spinal cord is situated within the vertebral canal of vertebral column and is surrounded by three meninges, namely, the duramater, the arachnoid, and the piamater. Further protection is provided by cerebrospinal fluid which surrounds the spinal cord in the subarachnoid space. Cord begins at the foramen magnum in the skull where it is continuous with the medulla oblongata of the brain. It terminates in the lumbar region.

Along the entire length of spinal cord are attached 31 pairs of spinal nerves by the ventral or motor roots and dorsal or sensory roots. Each dorsal nerve root possesses a dorsal root ganglion, the cells of which give rise to peripheral and central nerve fibers.

Brain: The brain is divided into three major divisions, namely, hind brain, mid brain, and forebrain.

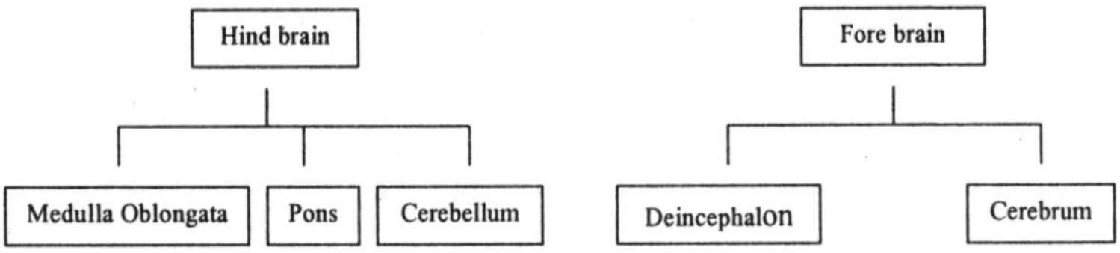

The brain stem (a collective term for the medulla oblongata, pons, and mid brain) is that part of the brain that remains after the cerebral hemispheres and cerebellum.

Major division of peripheral nervous system

The peripheral nervous system consists of the cranial and spinal nerves and their associated ganglia.

Cranial and spinal nerves

There are 12 pairs of cranial nerves which leave the brain and pass through different foramina in the skull. There are 31 pairs of spinal nerves which leave the spinal cord and pass through the intervertebral foramina in the vertebral column. The spinal nerves are named according to the region of the vertebral column with which they are associated. There are 8 pairs of cervical, 12 pairs of thoracic, 5 pairs of lumbar, 5 pairs of sacral, and one pair of coccygeal nerves (Fig. 1).

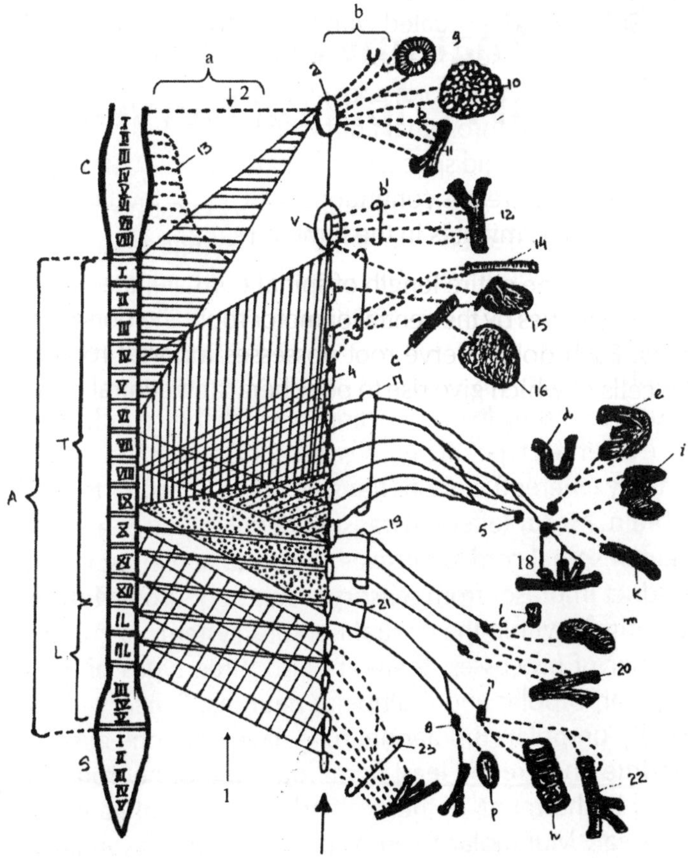

Fig. 1: Schematic drawing of sympathetic nervous system

A: Thoraco lumbar segment, C: Cervical, T: Thoracic, L: Lumbar & S: Sacral segments

1. Sympathetic trunk, 2. Cervical cranial ganglion, 3. Stellate ganglion, 4. Thoracic ganglion, 4′. Lumbar ganglion, 5. Solar plexus, 6. Renal and suprarenal plexus, 7. Caudal mesenteric plexus, 8. Hypogastric plexus, 9. Eye vessel, 10. Vessels of salivary gland, 11. Cranial vessel, 12. Cervical vessel, 13. Spinal nerve, 14. Vessels of forelimbs, 15. Heart, 16. Lung vessel, 17. Greater splanchnic nerve.18. Vessels of stomach, liver, spleen and intestine 19. Lesser splanchnic nerve 20. Vessels of kidneys and adrenal gland 21.Hypogastric nerve 22.Vessels of large intestine, urogenital organs 23. Vessels of hind limb; a. Preganglionic fibre b, postganglionic fibres (interrupted line), c. Trachea, d. Small intestine e. stomach, i. liver k. spleen, l. adrenal gland, m. kidney, n. large intestine, p. urinary bladder.

4 Anatomy and Physiology of Peripheral Nerves

The nervous system structures are mainly composed of two kinds of cells namely neurons and neuralgia. The **neurons** are specialized in impulse conduction. The **neuralgia,** the supporting tissue of central nervous system (brain and spinal cord) perform less specialized function, while most of the supporting tissue of the peripheral nervous system is ordinary white fibrous connective tissue. According to the direction in which they conduct impulses, there are three types of neurons, sensory, motor and interneurons. **Sensory** (afferent) neurons transmit nerve impulses to spinal cord or brain. **Motor** (efferent) transmit nerve impulses away from the brain or spinal cord to muscles or glandular tissues. Interneurons conduct impulses from sensory to motor neurons. **Interneurons** lie entirely within the central nervous system. According to the number of processes, there are also three types of neurons — unipolar, bipolar and multipolar neurons. Sensory neurons are usually unipolar. Bipolar neurons have only one axon and one dendrite and are the least numerous kind of neurons. They are found in the retina of the eye and in the spinal ganglion of the inner ear. Multipolar neurons have only one axon and several dendrites. Most of the neurons in the brain and spinal cord are multipolar. All neurons consist of a cell body and at least two processes; one axon and one or more dendrites. Because dendrites and axons are thread-like extensions from neuron's body, they are often called nerve fibers. **Dendrites** are short protoplasmic processes that branch repeatedly. The distal ends of dendrites of sensory neurons are called receptors because they receive the stimuli that initiate conduction. Dendrites conduct impulses to the cell body of the neuron. The axon of a neuron is a single process that extends out from the neuron's cell body. Axons vary in both the length and diameter. In general, the larger the diameter, the more rapid the conduction. A neuron's axon conducts impulses away from its cell body.

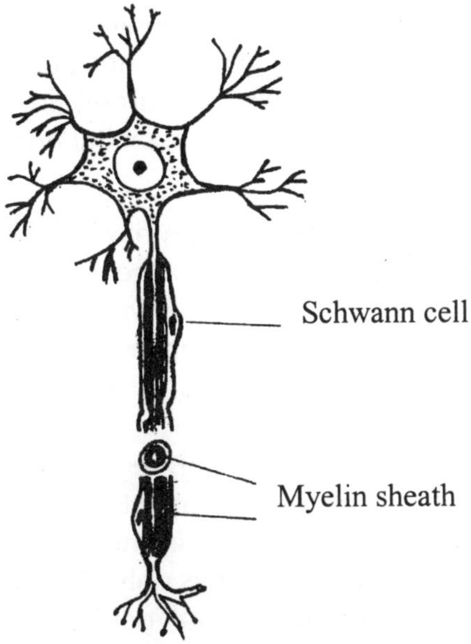

Fig. 2: Structure of a neuron

The **myelin sheath,** a fatty substance is a segmented wrapping around a nerve fiber. It is produced by either a **Schwann cell** and or **oligodendroglia** cell. To form the myelin sheath the Schwann cell wraps itself around the nerve fiber in jelly role fashion (Fig. 2). Oligodendroglia form the myelin sheaths around central nerve fibers, i.e., those located in the brain and spinal cord. Fibers that have a myelin sheath are called myelinated fibers, but those that have only a thin layer of myelin are called **unmyelinated fibers**. Because of the high fat content of myelin, bundles of myelinated fibers have a white creamy colour, and they make up the white matter of the nervous system. The bundles of myelinated fibers (axons) located in the brain and spinal cord are called as **tracts**. The bundles of myelinated fibers located outside the brain and spinal cord are called **nerves.**

The **neurollema**, sheath of Schwann consist of a Schwann cell wrapped once around a nerve fiber to form a continuous sheath enclosing the segmented myelin sheaths of peripheral nerve fibers. Brain and spinal cord fibers do not have a neurollema. Because the neurollema plays an essential role in the regeneration of cut or injured nerve fibers, peripheral nerve fibers regenerate but brain and cord fibers presumably do not. In unmyelinated fibers impulse travels along the axon as a localized propagating chemical change, surrounded by an electric field approximately spherically-oriented around the axon as a core, but in a myelinated fiber it cannot do so since the myelin acts as an insulator. Thus the ionic shifts that underlie the rising and falling phases of the action potential in myelinated fibers take place at the nodes, and in such fibers electric current flows not between immediately adjacent zones of the axon but from one **node of Ranvier** to the next.

Spinal nerves: They have no special name but are numbered according to the level of the spinal column at which they emerge from the spinal cavity. A typical spinal nerve has roots, the nerve proper and various branches (Fig. 3). The spinal nerve is a mixed nerve. Each spinal nerve, instead of attaching directly to the cord, attaches indirectly by means of two short roots, dorsal and ventral. The dorsal root is readily recognized by observing an enlargement at the place of attachment, the **dorsal root ganglion** or **spinal ganglion** which contains nerve cell bodies of afferent neurons. The dorsal root carries only afferent (sensory) impulses towards spinal cord. The ventral root contains efferent fibers and emerges from the ventral portion of the spinal cord. It carries efferent

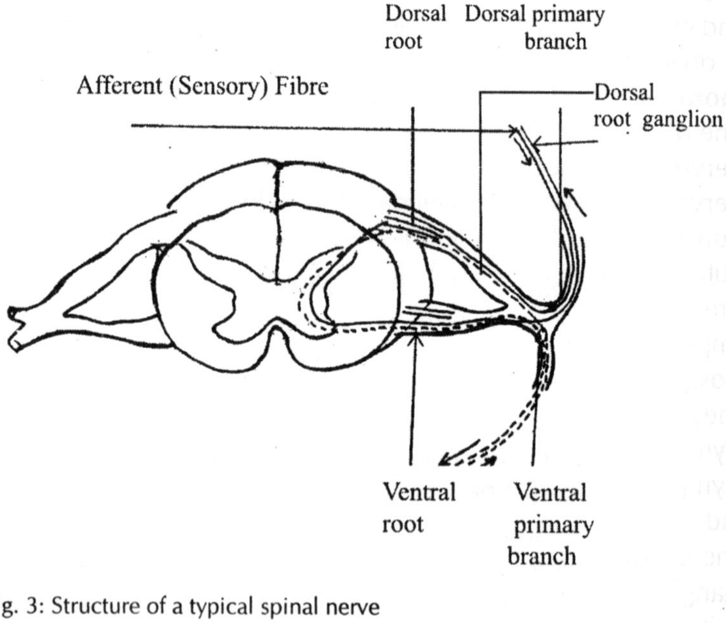

Fig. 3: Structure of a typical spinal nerve

(motor) impulses from the spinal cord to striated muscle fibers. The spinal nerve after leaving the intervertebral foramen divides into the dorsal and ventral branches which both contain sensory and motor fibers. The dorsal branches of the spinal nerves supply structures that are dorsal to the transverse processes of the vertebrae, e.g., the muscles and skin of the body, while the ventral branches supply the muscles and skin of the ventral aspect of chest and abdomen and fore and hind limbs. Each fore limb is supplied by a **brachial plexus**, which is a network of nerves formed by the union of the last three or four cervical and first one or two thoracic nerves. The spinal cord shows a considerable increase in size in this region known as the **cervical enlargement.** Each hind limb is supplied with **lumbosacral plexus,** which is made up of the ventral branches of the last few lumbar and first one or two sacral nerves.

The autonomic nervous system: The autonomic nervous system is composed of autonomic or visceral motor neurons (neurons that conduct impulses from the central nervous system to the visceral effectors, i.e., cardiac muscles, smooth muscles and glandular epithelial tissues). The autonomic nervous system is divided into the **craniosacral** or **parasympathetic** and the **thoracolumbar** or **sympathetic divisions.** The **hypothalamus** is one of the major areas of the brain that controls the autonomic nervous system. Both divisions consist of autonomic ganglia and nerves. Autonomic ganglia contain synapses and cell bodies of autonomic neurons. Autonomic nerves contain axons of autonomic neurons. Autonomic neurons are of two types namely, pre-ganglionic and postganglionic. **Preganglionic neurons** transmit impulses from the central nervous system to an autonomic neuron. **Postganglionic neurons** on the other hand, conduct impulses after they reach a ganglion, i.e., from a ganglion to a visceral effector. **Sympathetic ganglia** lie lateral to ventral surface of spinal column. Sympathetic division consists of two chains or ganglia on each side of the spinal column from the level of cervical vertebrae to the coccyx and are often referred to as the sympathetic chain ganglia. Short fibers connect each ganglion with each other and with thoracic and lumbar segments of cord; other fibers extend from sympathetic ganglia out to visceral effectors. The sympathetic pre-ganglionic neurons have their cell bodies in lateral gray columns of thoracic and first three or four segments of cord; axons leave cord in ventral roots of spinal nerves, leave spinal nerve by way of white ramus, and then follow one of the three paths; to terminate in sympathetic ganglia; or to and through sympathetic trunk to terminate in or lower sympathetic ganglia; or to and through sympathetic ganglia through splanchnic nerves to terminate in collateral ganglia (Fig. 1). Sympathetic postganglionic neurons have their dendrites and cell bodies in the sympathetic chain ganglia or in **collateral ganglia.** Their axons are distributed by both spinal nerves and separate autonomic nerves. They reach the spinal nerves via small filaments **(gray rami)** that connect the sympathetic ganglia with the spinal nerves. From the spinal nerves they travel to blood vessels, sweat glands, and erector hair muscles all over the body.

The parasympathetic preganglionic neurons have their cell bodies in nuclei of brain stem and of sacral segments of cord; axons from brain stem nuclei through cranial nerve VIII, in ciliary ganglion; from nuclei in pons through cranial nerve VII, terminate in sphinopalatine or submaxillary ganglion; from nuclei in medulla through cranial nerve IX to otic ganglion or through cranial nerves X and XI to cardiac and celiac ganglia. Parasympathetic postganglionic neurons have their dendrites and cell bodies in the outlying sympathetic ganglia or near organ innervated; axons lie in short nerves extending into effector.

The sympathetic division is chiefly an emergency system that greatly increases conduction to most visceral effectors during stress and prepares body for maximum energy expenditure and physical exertion by producing "fight or flight" reaction a group of sympathetic responses including increased epinephrine secretion by adrenal medulla, whereas the parasympathetic division regulates many visceral effectors under normal, everyday conditions; in general its neurotransmitter, acetylcholine, stimulate organ secretions and contraction of smooth muscle of digestive tract thereby increases peristalsis.

Excitation of plasma membrane of the nerve cell body:

When the nerve cell is excited (stimulated) by electrical, mechanical, or chemical means, a rapid change in membrane permeability to Na^+ ions take place and Na^+ ions diffuse through the plasma membrane into the cell cytoplasm from the tissue fluid. The sudden influx of Na^+ ions followed by the altered polarity produces action potential, which is approximately +40mV. This potential is very brief, lasting about 5 msec. followed by increased permeability for K^+ ion which starts to flow from the cell cytoplasm and return the localized area of the cell to the resting state. Once generated, the action potential spreads over the plasma membrane, away from the site of initiation and is conducted along neurites as the nerve impulse, which is self propagated and its size and frequency does not alter. Once the nerve impulse has spread over a given region of plasma membrane another action potential cannot be elicited immediately. The duration of this non-excitable state is referred to as the refractory period. Inhibitory stimuli are believed to produce their effect by causing an influx of Cl^- ions through the plasma membrane into the neuron, thus producing hyperpolarization and reducing the excitatory state of the cell.

5 Local Anaesthetics

Local anaesthetics are a group of drugs that reversibly block the propagation of action potentials along nerve axons. These are used to anaesthetize a region of the body. These agents are applied directly at the target site.

History

The first local anaesthetic was an alkaloid, cocaine, isolated from the leaves of South American shrub *Erythroxylon coca*, which produced a sense of well-being to allay hunger and fatigue (for native runners of the area). Gaedicke extracted erythroxylun from the leaves of the plant in 1855 and Niemann isolated cocaine in 1860.

The first use of cocaine as local anaesthetic was described by Peruvian army surgeon. Koeller in 1884 revealed that instillation of cocaine into conjunctival sac anaesthetized the eye which led to its use in ophthalmology as a local anaesthetic. This was used in dental and surgical procedures by method of infiltration and nerve blocking. In 1855 Corning injected cocaine

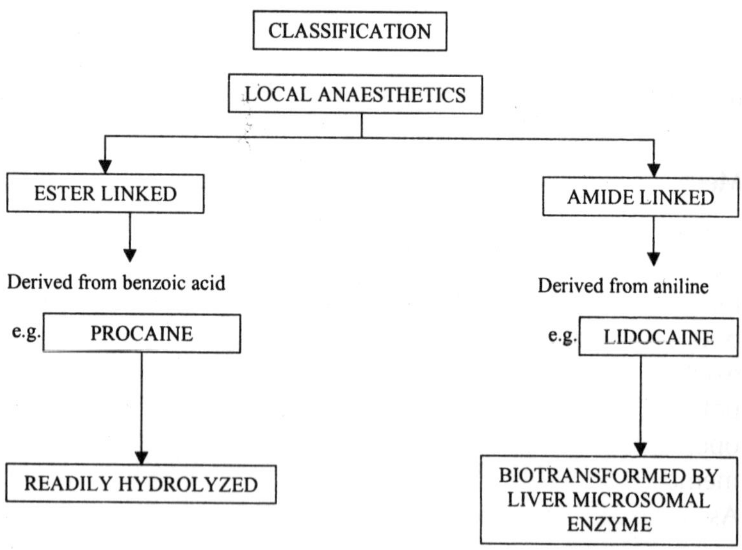

intrathecally. Also in 1855 Mclean used cocaine for nerve blocks of limbs in a horse. Willstatter in 1902 completed the structure and final synthesis of cocaine.

Classification

Local anaesthetics may be classified as Ester-linked or Amide-linked, depending on the structure of the molecules intermediate chain. Those derived from benzoic acid belong to ester family (e.g., procaine) and those derived from aniline belong to aminoacyl or amide family (e.g., lignocaine). The nature of intermediate chain predetermines the course of biotransformation.

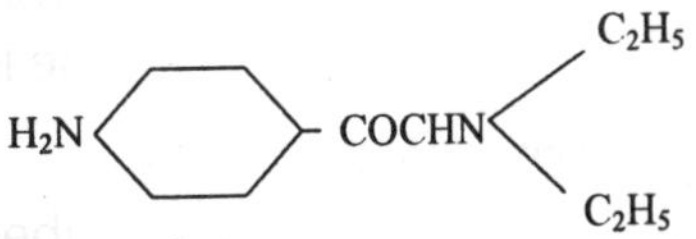

Procaine

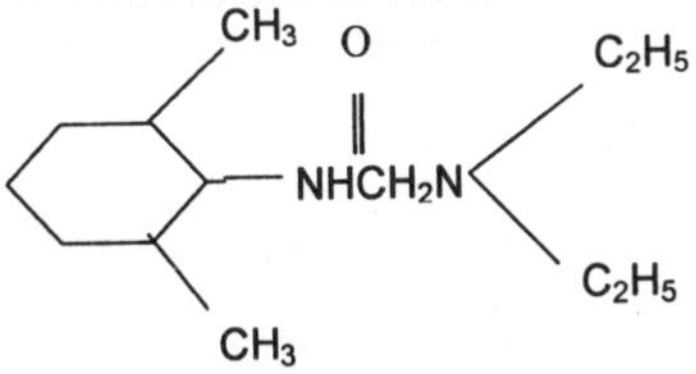

Lidocaine

Classification based on potency and duration

i) Low potency and short duration e.g., procaine, chlorocaine

ii) Intermediate potency and duration e.g., mepivacaine, prilocaine, lidocaine

iii) High potency and long duration e.g., tetracaine, bupivacaine, etidocaine

Mechanism of action

These agents prevent the rapid influx of Na^+ ions into nerve axons that produces the action potential. These act by binding to receptors located on Na^+ channels. Local anaesthetics prevent both generation and the conduction of nerve impulse. The excitable membrane of nerve axons maintains a transmembrane potential of 90 to 60 mV. During excitation, the sodium channels open and a fast inward sodium current quickly depolarizes the membrane towards the sodium equilibrium potential (+40mV). As a result of depolarization, the sodium channels close (inactivate) and potassium channels open. The outward flow of K^+ repolarizes the membrane towards the potassium equilibrium potential (-95mV); repolarization returns the sodium channels to the rested state. The transmembrane ionic gradients are maintained by the sodium pump. When increasing concentrations of a local anaesthetic are applied to a nerve fiber, the threshold for excitation increases, the impulse conduction slows, the rate of rise of the action potential declines. The action potential amplitude decreases and finally, the ability to generate an action potential is abolished. All these effects result from the binding of the local anaesthetic to sodium channels/receptors which in turn block the transient permeability to sodium. If the sodium current is blocked over a critical portion of nerve, propagation of an impulse over the blocked area is no longer possible.

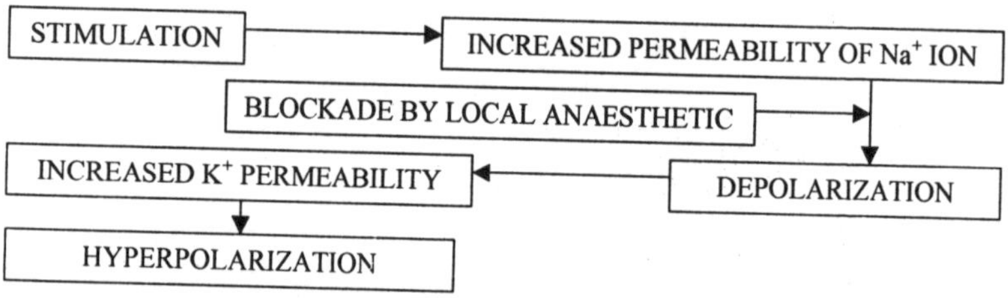

Pharmacokinetics

Absorption is influenced by many factors, including dosage (volume and concentration), site of injection, presence of vasoconstrictor substance (Adrenaline) and physicochemical and pharmacological properties of the drug. Local anaesthetic deposited in a highly vascular area will be absorbed more rapidly and attain higher blood levels than if injected into tissue of less blood flow. The presence of vasoconstrictor tends to reduce systemic absorption by reducing local blood flow.

Distribution: Amide local anaesthetic agents are widely distributed in the body. Distribution of ester anaesthetics is much more limited because their plasma half lives are very short. Protein binding also influences plasma drug concentration.

Biotransformation and excretion: The esters are primarily

hydrolyzed by plasma pseudocholinesterase, whereas amides undergo enzymatic degradation in liver. Cocaine is an atypical ester because it undergoes significant hepatic metabolism and urinary excretion. A common pathway in biotransformation of amide local anaesthetics is dealkylation which occurs within hepatic microsomes.

These are excreted from the body via urine or bile. The majority of p-amino benzoic acid formed after procaine metabolism is excreted unchanged as a conjugated product in the urine. In general, because most local anaesthetics contain alkaline amino radicals, excretion in an acid urine is greater because of increased ionization. In alkaline urine, renal elimination of local anaesthetic is delayed or slowed because the drug remains principally in the unionized state and may be reabsorbed.

6 Pharmacological Properties and Mechanism of Action of Local Analgesics

Most injectable local analgesics are tertiary amines. A few are secondary amines. The general configuration of a local anaesthetic is composed of two key-structural components: one imparting a lipid solubility (lipophilic) and the other imparting water solubility (hydrophilic). These two components are joined by an intermediate hydrocarbon chain, which is usually either an ester or an amide linkage. Compounds that lack the hydrophilic portion of the molecule are almost insoluble in water and therefore, not suitable for injection, but they are frequently used in topical anaesthesia of mucous membranes (e.g., benzocaine).

Local analgesics are weak bases with a dissociation constant (pK) between 7 and 10. Because they are poorly soluble and unstable in water, they are usually clinically available as the water soluble acid salt. Local anaesthetic agents that are generally water soluble acid salts that dissociate on hydrolysis into active agents in neutral and alkaline areas. They are not effective in an acid medium (e.g., abscess). This is confirmed clinically, when local anaesthetic is injected into tissues having an acid medium due to accumulation of pus that prevents hydrolysis of the acid salt and the freeing of potent alkaloidal base. This is the reason, why an abscessed area is impossible or difficult to anaesthetize thoroughly. When injected into the tissues that normally are slightly alkaline, the acid salt from the local anaesthetic is neutralized. This releases the amine or alkaloidal base through hydrolysis, which is necessary before it can penetrate the lipid barrier of the cell membrane to induce anaesthesia. The degree of ionization of the molecule is determined by the pK and pH of the tissues. When the pH of the solution is the same as the pK of the anaesthetic drug, half the drug exists as the cation and the other half as the base. Apparently only the base form can penetrate the nerve membrane. Alkalization of local anaesthetic solution speeds the onset and effectiveness of a block, *albeit* rendering the solution too unstable for clinical practice. The buffer reserve in normal tissue tends to maintain a constant pH delaying neutralization and therefore, full effect of the local analgesia. Anaesthesia might be inadequate in inflammed tissues because of low pH of the interstitial fluid, causing reduced liberation of free anaesthetic base. Local anaesthetic solution must diffuse from the site of injection to the nerve and penetrate fibers and connective tissue before reaching the individual axons within the nerve. Intraneural diffusion then continues from the nerve mantle to the core, as manifested clinically by nerve blocks spreading from proximal to distal parts of the body. Recovery of function occurs in the same order when the analgesic solution is effectively exhausted by dilution with tissue fluids, dispersion away from the nerve, uptake by the blood stream, and metabolic inactivation. The latency depends upon nerve diameter, pH, diffusion rate, and anaesthetic concentration. The higher the concentration of the analgesic solution, the more rapid is the onset of the block.

Local anaesthetic agents prevent the generation and propagation of the nerve impulse. Their main site of action is the cell membrane, as they interfere with its permeability to sodium. They decrease the permeability of the cell membrane and stabilize the membrane forces by combining amino groups of local analgesics like procaine, with polar group of cell membrane. As a result diffusion of sodium and potassium ions cannot occur, thus the changes that create nerve impulse are blocked. Another mechanism of local anaesthetic action involves the action of these agents upon the membrane calcium. Both calcium and local analgesics have stabilizing effect upon excitable membrane, that is indicated by the fact that both calcium and local anaesthetic increase the threshold of electric stimulation of the membrane, thus the nerve impulse conduction is blocked without any change in the resting membrane potential. It is believed that local anaesthetic agents act by interfering with the ionic conduction, particularly of calcium ions, which in turn checks the catecholamine release, thereby preventing stimulation. Increased calcium concentration in the medium bathing the nerve may either relieve or intensify conduction block produced by local analgesics. Relief occurs because calcium alters the surface potential on the membrane. Calcium may also intensify the degree of conduction block by altering the kinetics of opening the sodium channel.

All anaesthetic agents including local analgesics result in deformation or expansion of cell membrane. Binding of local anaesthetic molecule to hydrophobic regions of cell membrane and expansion of some critical regions in the membrane may also prevent increased sodium ion permeability thereby stopping propagation of an action potential or nerve-impulse conduction. Another interesting mechanism regarding local anaesthetic is flow of sodium ions. According to this, the sodium channels are surrounded by ring-like structures formed by lipid molecules that are in a crystalline or jell state. Rigidity of these channels permits the flow of sodium ions. Local analgesics are believed to reduce the rigidity of these channels and change them from solid to liquid crystalline state. This closes the channels to sodium ion thus depolarization cannot occur and anaesthesia is induced.

A local anaesthetic produces a depolarizing block that takes effect at the surface membrane of excitable tissue cells. Smooth and striated muscles (blood vessels and myocardium) as well as nerve fibers are effected. The site of action of a local anaesthetic in a myelinated nerve is at the node of Ranvier, and 2 to 3 adjacent nodes must be exposed to the local anaesthetic to prevent saltatory conduction. At least 6 mm and preferably 1 cm of nerve length be exposed to anaesthetic solution to deter impulses from bypassing the blockade segments. Nerve conduction is interrupted because generation of an action potential is prevented by obstruction of the inward flow of sodium ions through the nerve membranes. A low concentration of local anaesthetic may simply delay the migration of ions without completely preventing it. The electrical excitability of myocardial tissue is reduced by agents such as lidocaine or procainamide, which hinder the transmission of stimuli and inhibit the appearance of ectopic foci. In central nervous system, it has been demonstrated that a sub-convulsive dose of lidocaine can have an anticonvulsant effect due to its stabilizing properties on excitable membrane. There are three main types of nerve fibers, A, B, and C. Myelinated somatic nerve fibers are classified as 'A' fibers and subdivided into alpha, beta, gamma and delta, according to decreasing chain and conduction velocity. Alpha fibers are the largest and most rapidly conducting; delta fibers are the smallest and slowest conducting. B fibers are myelinated autonomic Preganglionic fibers. C fibers are nonmyelinated easily blocked fibers, both somatic and autonomic. Local anaesthetic agents block the fibers in the following order, B, C, delta, gamma, beta and alpha fibers. Recovery occurs in the reverse order. Compression of a nerve on the contrary, block A fibers, alpha and beta groups, subserve motor function, proprioception and touch; small A fibers the delta group and C fibers subserve pain and temperature sensation.

7 Clinically Common Local Analgesics

Ester linked

Procaine hydrochloride: It was synthesized by Einhorn in 1904 and introduced in 1905 under the trade name of 'novocain' after cocaine was discovered to be habit-forming and relatively toxic. Procaine is less toxic and is rapidly hydrolyzed in plasma. Therefore the analgesia produced is relatively brief. Analgesia with prociane is commonly prolonged by the addition of a vasoconstrictor to the solution to delay absorption of the local analgesic from the site of injection. This was the first of the synthetic true local analgesics and until the advent of lignocaine was considered the best for routine veterinary use. Compared to cocaine its power of penetration of mucous membranes is poor and hence is ineffective topically. It is almost non-irritant to tissues. Solutions of procaine can be sterilized by boiling. Procaine is decomposed by alkali. It is an inexpensive, relatively safe local anaesthetic used often for general infiltration in the dog and cat, as 2% solution combined with 1:1,00,000 adrenaline hydrochloride. In cattle and horses for skin infiltration and perineural injection 2.5% solution is effective. Anaesthesia is present in about 5 minutes and in case of epidural and perineural injection in about 10 minutes, and persists for about an hour. The maximal safe dose for an animal may be up to 1000 mg, provided absorption is reasonably slow. The anaesthetic solutions, of which procaine hydrochloride is the active principle, are chlorocaine, kerocaine, planocaine, and novutux.

Tetracaine hydrochloride (pontocaine): It was first synthesized in 1928. Tetracaine, like procaine, is an ester of p-aminobenzoic acid, and it is hydrolyzed by plasma cholinesterase. It is approximately 10 times more toxic than procaine. Because of its longer duration of action, it is still one of the preferred agents for the conduction and spinal anaesthesia. It is an optimal topical anaesthetic for the eye at a concentration of 0.5% in small animals and 1% in large animals. A concentration of 2% is used to produce surface anaesthesia of mucous membranes. Veterinary ophthalmologists seldom use tetracaine on the eye in surgical procedures because it appears to delay post-surgical wound healing.

Proparacaine hydrochloride (opthaine): It is an ester-linked topical anaesthetic. It has a potency similar to or slightly greater than that of tetracaine and is available as a 0.5% solution. The surface anaesthesia develops within 1 minute after its topical use and its effect lasts for about 15 minutes. One drop of a 0.5% solution is recommended at 5 to 10 minutes interval for 5 to 7 times in cataract surgery. It has also been used for topical anaesthesia of the nose and ear, for wound management and prior to catheterization. It is currently the topical agent of choice for corneal anaesthesia.

Amide linked

Lignocaine hydrochloride (lidocaine): It was synthesized in 1943 and first used in Sweden. Chemically, it is an alkyl amine derivative of meta-xylene (dimethyl-benzene). Lignocaine is very stable and probably the most widely used agent by all routes of administration. It can also be used for ophthalmic purpose. It can be boiled with strong acids or alkalis for several hours without decomposing. Compared with procaine, lignocaine has a far shorter period of onset, a more intense and a longer duration of action. Being a very effective local anaesthetic, it has replaced almost all local analgesics. It has great penetrating power, excellent topical action as 4% solution, is used for surface anaesthesia of mucous membranes particularly those of throat and larynx before endotracheal intubation. It is very useful for epidural and plexus blocks (0.5 to 2% solutions). It has marked central effects, including drowsiness, sedation. Nerve blocks are optimally performed with 1.5 to 2% solution with the addition of epinephrine (1:2,00,000). The dose for epidural anaesthesia in dogs is 1 ml/5 kg of 2% solution with adrenaline 1:1,00,000. In horses and cattle 10 to 12 ml of 2% solution can be used without the onset of inco-ordination of the rear limbs. In cats, 2 ml of 2% solution with 1:1,00,000 adrenaline is used. Maximal safe dose is 200 mg without and 500 mg with the addition of epinephrine. The approximate maximum dose by infiltration before toxic signs become apparent is not known with any certainty but is thought to be of the order of 10 mg/kg. Liver is the only tissue that has been shown to metabolize lignocaine in significant quantities. All amide-linked local anaesthetic agents are almost completely metabolized by the liver before excretion.

Bupivacaine hydrochloride (marcain): It was synthesized in 1957. Bupivacaine is dl-1-butyl-2′,6′-pipecoloxylidide hydrochloride. Bupivacaine is a very stable compound and shows no change on repeated autoclaving. It is a highly lipid soluble substance. It is approximately 4 times more potent than lignocaine, hence 0.5% solution is equivalent in nerve blocking activity to a 2 % solution of lignocaine. The addition of adrenaline in low concentration has been shown to increase both the speed of onset and the duration of anaesthesia so that all solutions of bupivacaine available for clinical use contain adrenaline. It has longer latency but is considerably longer lasting. It possesses, to greater or lesser degrees, the most desirable general properties of a local analgesic drug. It is generally agreed that bupivacaine provides a period of analgesia at least twice as long as that of lignocaine, and that it is exceptionally well tolerated by all tissues. It is one of the agents of choice for continuous epidural anaesthesia. The comparatively long duration of action is a valuable characteristic for situations where prolonged anaesthesia is required. The maximal safe dose is 2 mg/kg of body weight in animals.

Mepivacaine hydrochloride (carbocaine): It is an amide-linked local aneasthetic that was synthesized in 1956. It has the equivalent potency of lignocaine. It is slightly less toxic than lignocaine but its action is longer even without adrenaline. A 1% solution with adrenaline (1:200000) has been recommended for epidural anaesthesia in dogs at a dose rate of 0.5 ml every 30 seconds and was continued until the toe reflexes disappeared, indicating that surgical analgesia up to T_5 has been attained. It has also been used for topical anaesthesia of equine larynx. A 2% solution has been especially found useful for equine nerve blocks, because there is less post- injection edema than with lignocaine.

Prilocaine hydrochloride (citanest): It is available in 1%, 2% and 3% concentrations for injections. It is amide linked and resembles lignocaine chemically. The onset and duration of action are longer than lignocaine. Similar to the action of lignocaine, prilocaine may also produce drowsiness. Once the dose of prilocaine exceeds therapeutic levels, it leads to complications. Five ml 2% prilocaine has been administered in sheep intrathecally and epidurally. Its anaesthetic effect varied from 39 to 69 minutes. It shows a good promise to be used for all types of infiltrations and regional nerve blocks as well as for spinal aneasthesia in animals. It is popular in equine surgery because it is said to produce less tissue reaction than lignocaine. It is the most rapidly metabolized amide and its metabolism releases o-toluidine which causes methaemoglobinaemia. However, the extent or degree of the methaemoglobinaemia apparently is of little consequence provided therapeutic levels are not exceeded.

8 Local Analgesic Techniques

Surface or topical analgesia: Surface or topical analgesia is produced when local anaesthetic drugs are applied or introduced to surfaces capable of absorption since un-abraded skin surfaces limits their penetration. Local analgesics diffuse through the mucous surfaces to cause loss of sensation by paralysing nerve endings. Many a times local analgesics are combined with other therapeutic agents in a cream or jelly form to provide relief in clinical cases like dermatitis, pruritis and otitis externa, conjunctivitis in animals. A topical application of 2% lignocaine in carboxymethyl cellulose gel is frequently used to anaesthetise and lubricate mucous surfaces as it has good local anaesthetic effect. This is generally employed for nasal, lacrimal, endotracheal and urethral catheterization and for otic examination. It has been used for the relief of pain in the mucous membranes of the mouth, pharynx, larynx, vulva and glans penis. A topical application of 2% viscous lidocaine facilitates intubation in anaesthetised dogs. Opthaine (proparacaine hydrochloride) is the agent of choice for surface analgesia of conjunctiva and cornea for minor ophthalmic surgery. This compound does not produce pupilary dilatation and is non-irritant, but its solution is rather unstable, having a shelf-life of only 12 months. The local anaesthetic solution is also injected for therapeutic reasons into the urethra of animals suffering from obstruction due to calculi. It induces surface analgesia of urethra that relieves spasm and facilitates passage of stones.

Surface or topical analgesics are used for anaesthetising synovial membrane of joints and tendon sheaths for relief of pain arising from pathological processes. A solution of local anaesthetic agent is injected into the synovial cavity and then dispersed throughout the cavity by manipulation of the limb. If the synovial cavity is distended with fluid, it is first drained to ensure that the injected solution is not excessively diluted. The injection renders synovial membrane insensitive within 5 to 10 minutes and the effect persists for about an hour. The intra-articular injection of local analgesic is also employed to aid diagnosis of lameness (Fig. 4). Clearly, almost every joint and tendon sheath in the body can be treated in this way. A needle can be introduced into synovial sheaths quite easily when they are distended with synovial fluid, but entry into a normal sheath is not easy. However, as soon as the needle enters the sheath the resistance to injection disappears and some of the solution enters the synovial cavity, lifting its wall away from the underlying tendon.

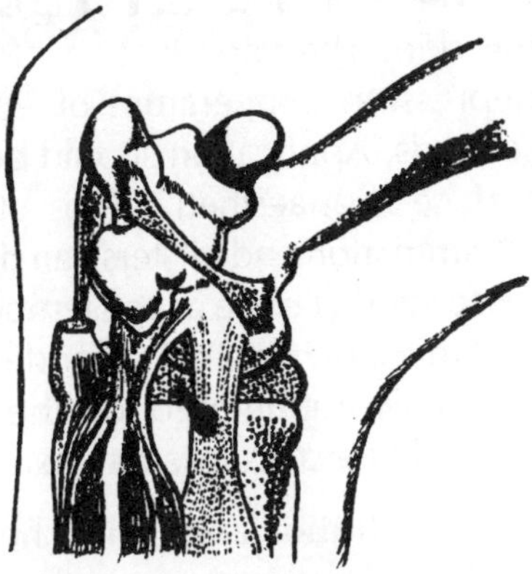

Fig. 4: Approach to the lateral sac of the femorotibial joint between the lateral fumorotibial ligament and the common tendon of the long digital extensor and the peroneus tertius

The topical anaesthetic effective on the intact skin is now available which is an eutectic mixture of lignocaine and prilocaine (1:1). The melting point of the mixture is lower than that of individual drugs and the combination is liquid at room temperature. A cream made from this mixture has been used for anaesthesia of intact skin.

Analgesia by freezing: It is a form of surface analgesia that is produced by freezing agents. The analgesia produced by freezing agents is called **refrigeration analgesia.** It is used for small incisions, opening of abscesses and similar minor interferences as well as for routine injection in particularly sensitive animals. Ice is the simplest but generally volatile substances which cause freezing by the rapid volatilization from the surface of the skin are used. Ethyl chloride spray, ether spray and carbonic acid snow are examples. Their action is very superficial and transient. The skin may advantageously be sprayed with ethyl chloride. The drug is directed from 30 cm distance on the skin. The vaporization of the drug, which has a maximal depression temperature of -35° C, freezes the skin in a few seconds. Application should be stopped immediately, once the surface is anaesthetized, as otherwise damage in the form of inflammation and blisters can develop. The interference must be performed at once as the temporary insensitivity only persists 1 to 2 minutes. As ethyl chloride vapour is very inflammable, this drug may not be used together with the electrocautery or near fires and electric installations.

Infiltration analgesia: The nerve endings are anaesthetised by their direct exposure to the drug at the actual site of incision. Except the digits and teats most minor surgical operations can be performed under infiltration anaesthesia. For major operation in animals, which are bad operative risk, this type of anaesthesia can be given with light basal narcosis. Infiltration should, however, never be carried out through or into infected or inflamed tissues. Since lignocaine Hcl has better spreading power, it is used in the concentration of 0.2 to 0.5%. It is advisable to add adrenaline (1:40,000 or 1:200,000) to the solution, however vasoconstrictor should be avoided in situations where circulation of blood is interfered.

The limits of the area to be infiltrated are conveniently defined and marked by the use of intradermal weals. The intradermal weal is performed with the help of short needle that is held parallel to the skin surface with the bevel of its point uppermost away from the skin. A short (2 cm) needle is held almost parallel to the skin at 20° angle and thrust into the skin until the bevel is no longer visible. In large animals 1 to 2 ml and in small animals 0.3 to 0.5 ml of local anaesthetic solution is injected by exerting considerable pressure on the plunger of the syringe. The resulting weal is insensitive when it is formed. If punctures are repeatedly made at the periphery of such weals, a continuous weal can be produced along the proposed line of incision. Such intra-dermal infiltration is only easily performed in thick-skinned animals. In large animals like horses and cattle, the weal is raised at either end of the proposed line of infiltration. Subcutaneous tissues are infiltrated by introducing a needle (10 cm long) through skin at the site of the intradermal weal. Before injecting any local anaesthetic solution, aspiration is attempted to ascertain that the needle point has not entered a blood vessel. To infiltrate several layers of tissue, such as those that form the abdominal wall, the procedure is to inject, from one puncture site, first the subcutaneous tissue and then, in succession by further advancing the needle, the musculature, the intervening connective tissue, and so on to the full depth. About 1 ml of solution is required for every centimeter of incision. If the proposed site of incision is longer than the needle, it is introduced through a weal in the centre of the site and directed first in one direction and then in the opposite direction.

Field block: This is attained by desensitizing an area by infiltration of its margins. It consists of making walls of analgesia enclosing the operative field. It is achieved by making fan-wise injections in certain planes of the body to soak all the nerves that cross these planes on their way to the operative field, but no attempt is made to pick out the nerves individually. Usually the entire thickness of the soft tissue in which the nerves run is involved. The advantage is that the tissue around the actual incision is not infiltrated by anaesthetic solution and so remains unaltered and free from distortion. The healing of the wound is also not interfered. Operations involving the skin alone require only subcutaneous infiltration. This may be done from any two puncture sites. Operative fields involving deeper structures are blocked by infiltration in a sort of cup formation from two or more cutaneous sites. Generally, walls of analgesia are created obliquely to the skin surface, involving only part of the tissue around the region, but meeting below so that the operative area is held in a sort of cup of infiltrated tissue (Fig. 5). In veterinary practice field block commonly employed is that for rumenotomy. This block differs from the type of field block described above. Because of the course and distribution of the nerves supplying the operative site, it is usually produced by two linear infiltrations of the whole thickness of the body wall, one anterior to, and one above the line of incision in the form of inverted 'L' and the like patterns according to the need. The injection sites are the entire length of the posterior border of the last rib and along a line ventral to the transverse processes from the last rib to L_4. Also 2 to 4 inch area under L_4 should be injected (Fig. 6).

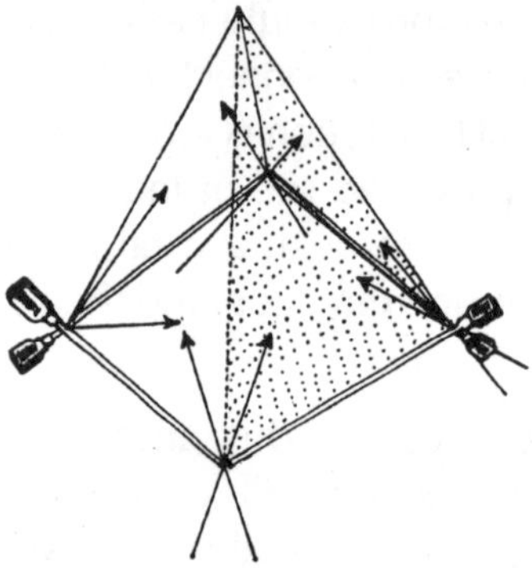

Fig. 5: Technique of field block (Production) of a cup of infiltrated tissue

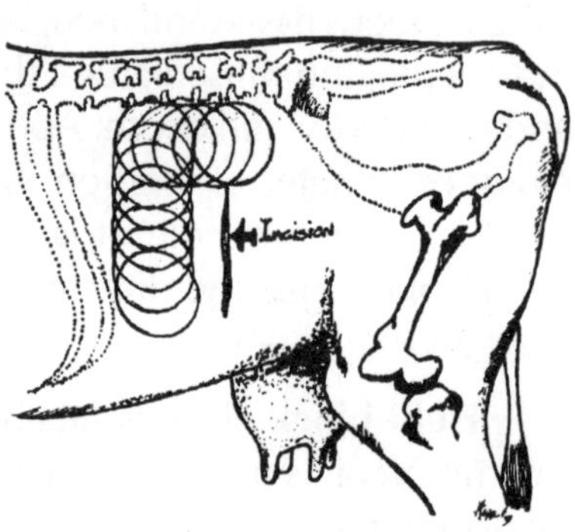

Fig. 6: Inverted "L." Block in cattle

Ring block: of an extremity is another special type of field block in which a transverse plane through the whole extremity is infiltrated with local anaesthetic solution and particular attention is given to the sites of large nerve trunks. Here peripheral circular infiltration of the extremity is performed. The technique is more effective when the injection is made distal to a tourniquet. The limb distal to the site is insensitive after about 15 minutes. One particular indication for peripheral infiltration is ring block of the metacarpus above the accessory digits for amputation of a digit in cattle. It is very useful in the fore limb, whereas

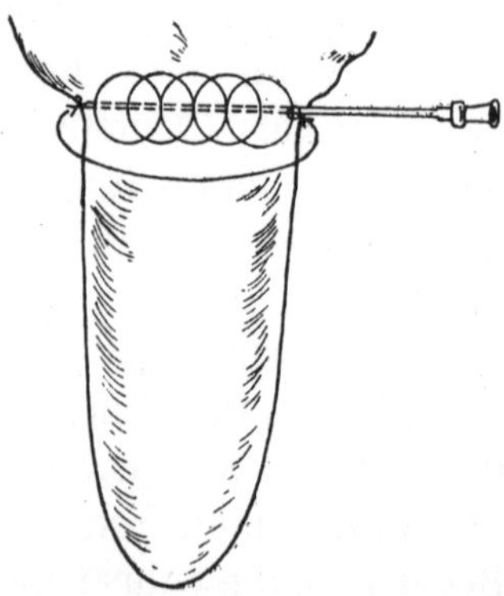

Fig. 7: Needle placement for ring block in a teat of cow

in hind quarters, epidural anaesthesia is more suitable. It may also be used for operations on cow's teats. Vasoconstrictors should not be added to the solution used to produce ring block in teats (Fig. 7) as prolonged vasoconstriction may result in ischaemic necrosis of the end of the teat.

9 Therapeutic Local Anaesthetic Blocks

The local anaesthetic agent procaine hydrochloride has also been used for therapeutic purposes in animals. In order to relieve spasmodic colic in horses, a solution of 0.5% procaine hydrochloride at the rate of 0.6 to 0.8 ml/kg, intravenously has been found effective. It has also been used for intestinal cramps in horses and colic in cattle. Sympathetic trunk and splanchnic nerves have been anaesthetised by introducing 0.5% procaine hydrochloride in the epipleural tissue at the level of last rib in horses and cattle. Epipleural block has been used in the treatment of spasmodic colic, gastro-enteritis, cystitis, peritonitis, hepatitis, metritis and nephritis in horses and cattle. It is also used as visceral anaesthesia for gastrotomy, cystotomy and enterotomy in dogs and sheep.

Epipleural blockade chiefly acts on nervous system, attenuating or suppressing irritation and inflammation. The organic and systemic functions remain normal. The thoracic procaine blockade technique is used in the treatment of bronchopneumonia in cattle. Procaine 0.5% at the rate of 0.5 ml/kg is administered at the level of 4th inter-costal space, that blocked the sympathetic trunks and their branches that resulted in the disappearance of the symptoms of bronchopneumonia. It is also used in the treatment of diarrhoea in calves with 0.5 to 1% procaine solution at the rate of 6 to 15 mg/kg body weight intra-peritoneally.

Blockade of splanchnic nerve and sympathetic trunk is found to anaesthetize the abdominal organs and it adequately relaxes the abdominal musculature. It has been used to delay premature parturition in cows and in cases of acute tympanites.

Intra-abdominal diffusion of procaine HCl results in its immediate absorption by peritoneum and the mesentery and results in visceral procaine anaesthesia, which facilitates abdominal surgery. In order to understand it, the following points should be borne in mind.

1. The somatic nervous system receives impulses from every site, including innervation of vegetative neurons and neurons themselves. Nerve centres affect the vegetative nervous system according to information received. The nervous system is permanently informed as to disposition of sympathetic and parasympathetic segments of vegetative nervous system. According to information gathered, its nervous centres influence the vegetative nervous system via central efferent neurons and their preganglionic nerve fibres, contacting with neurons of the vegetative nervous system and, therefore they control, co-ordinate and integrate its function according to adaptive requirements of the organism. The vegetative nervous system influences the functional state of nerve centres and periphery of the somatic nervous system by the principle of direct and reciprocal relations.
2. Sympathetic nerves are available in all organs innervated by cranial and parasympathetic nerves.
3. Every internal organ including cardiovascular system, are exposed to double "antagonistic" innervation by sympathetic and parasympathetic segments of the vegetative nervous system. This antagonism determines reciprocal inhibition, i.e., inhibition occurring in the parasympathetic segment, depression leads to reduction and simultaneous stimulation of sympathetic segment. These are attended by increase of tone of blood vessel walls and as a result, their lumen constricts and blood supply of the organs is thus impaired. But in contrast, inhibition of sympathetic is associated with promotion of functional activity of the organ and of blood circulation in these is enhanced.
4. All processes occurring in the body are under neurohumoral tropic influence that governs metabolism and ensures structure and function of tissues and organs that are inherent to them. Tropic influence exerted on tissues and organs is rendered by whole nervous system. But it is most pronounced

in sympathetic part of the vegetative nervous system that was assigned an adaptive tropic role. Due to impulses of this segment physicochemical changes occur in tissues presented as fundamental properties such as excitability, mobility, rapidity of response, etc.

5. Extent of response of organ and tissue stimulation are determined by fundamental influence of sympathetic segment, its reciprocal relationship to the parasympathetic segment and by conjugate (acting by the principle of direct and reciprocal relationship) interaction with somatic nervous system and endocrine glands (acting on the basis of direct and feedback relations). Moreover, impulse influence of sympathetic and parasympathetic nervous system affects secretory function of endocrine glands, while their hormones influence peripheral nervous structures like mediators, ensuring transmission of stimuli to peripheral working organs and cellular prostaglandins that stimulate specific response of cells of various organs. The functioning of the vegetative nervous system is constantly co-ordinated and integrated by brain stem.
6. It is known that strong and, especially, excessively strong stimuli affecting some site of the nerve lead to PARABIOSIS. The parabiotic site of the nerve does not conduct impulses, coming from extero-and intero-receptors to nerve centres and back. But excitability is very high at the site of the nerve that is adjacent to its parabiotic site. As a consequence, incessant torrent of strong stimuli travels from the excited site of the nerve to nerve centres, resulting in excitation and subsequent over-stimulation and parabiotic state of individual nerve centres and cerebral cortex. This is accompanied by impairment of adaptive tropic regulation of the periphery and internal organs and results in neuro-dystrophic symptoms, primarily in the pathological site.
7. Antiparabiotic effect is shown by procaine, direct current, anode, divalent cations of alkaline-earth material (Ca, Ba), adrenaline, infra-red rays, etc. Antiparabiotic factors make

conductance in the parabiotized nerve normal, reducing or completely reversing parabiosis. It should be remembered, however, that functional state of over-excited nerve, selected segments of the nervous system and its centres can also be normalised by parabiotic factors of mild stimulation, prescribed cooling, weak cathodic current, etc.

For therapeutic purpose, weak solutions of procaine (0.25 to 0.5%) are used, as they have antiparabiotic effect, that of 0.25% procaine being most prominent. Apart from antiparabiotic effect, procaine solutions have a certain chemotherapeutic action. Procaine is hydrolysed by tissue enzymes and blood serum, producing diethyl aminoethanol and para-amino banzoic acid (PABA). Having anti-histamine effect, the latter aids in reducing vessel permeability and inflammatory response, while diethyl aminoethanol improves circulation in the pathological site, moderately dilating the vessels.

High concentrations of procaine solution (2% and stronger) deepen parabiosis caused by pathological process and therefore do not yield therapeutic pathogenetic effect, but they do produce profound anaesthesia.

Therapeutic effect of procaine blockade (mechanism of action): the strong stimuli induce an impairment of tropic innervation and lead to neurodystrophy and domination of destructive component of inflammation over regeneration of reparative one, which becomes manifested a hyperegic inflammatory reaction, aggravation progress of disease. The replacement of strong stimulation of nervous system with weak one leads to normalisation of tropic enervation, and reduces or eliminates neurodystrophy. As a result, regenerative-reparative component becomes prevalent over destructive one in the inflammation focus over destructive one and the disease acquires benign course. Procaine blockade of the nerve and its receptors that are overexcited because of altering influences reduces or terminates the torrent of strong and excessively strong stimuli coming into nerve centres, replacing them by weak stimuli, coming from the site where local anaesthetic has been applied.

This reverses over-excitation of cerebral cortex, subcortical centres and reticular formation and, therefore, their tropic influence on the periphery and internal organs in improved. As a result, therapeutic effect of procaine blockade of pathologic focus is determined not by inhibition of receptors, nerves and other conduction pathways, but is due to improvement of their functional properties after blockade. Hence procaine solutions of weak concentrations, preferably 0.25% ought to be used for procaine blockades. Solutions stronger than 0.5% cause inhibition of conductance, persistent and complete analgesia effect.

It should be taken into account, however, that therapeutic effect of procaine blockade is determined by initial condition of somatic and vegetative nervous system, i.e., it depends on the degree of their over-stimulation (phase of parabiosis). In very severe pathological processes, attended by excessively strong stimulation of the nervous system, procaine blockade as additional nerve stimulation can render negative effect on the periphery, and even cause tissue necrosis.

Since there is reciprocal relationship between the parasympathetic and the sympathetic, it should be borne in mind that procaine blockade of either of them produces physiologically variable effect, just as procaine blockade of reflexogenic zones where the two segments form nerve plexuses, e.g., solar plexus and others. Procaine blockade of selective ranges of sympathetic segment of the vegetative nervous system is known to produce better improvement of tissue tropism and enhancement of regenerative-reparative processes. The strong or incessant prolonged stimuli coming from the periphery or internal organs are reduced or terminated under the influence of procaine blockade of somatic and particularly, vegetative conduction pathway and ganglia. This effect of blockade is primarily determined by termination of the torrent of strong stimuli into subcortical centres and cerebral cortex and by prolonged influence of procaine on peripheral nerve structures at the site of blockade and prolonged contact of procaine with various segments of the central nervous system.

Therefore, it is conceivable that prolonged influence of procaine on nerve centres, in particular on cerebral cortex, induces reduction or liquidation of foci of excitation. After procaine blockade coordinating influence of the cortex on reticular formation is restored and tonic effect on hypothalamus is reduced due to it. The latter exerts normalizing influence on the axis "pituitary-adrenal cortex". All these cause improvement of protective-adaptive responses and normalisation of tropic influence of nerve centres. With this blood circulation, intracellular and systemic metabolism are improved, capillary permeability, especially that at pathologic focus, is decreased, reticular endothelial system, phagocytosis and other immunologic responses are activated, neurodystrophy is improved, regenerative-reparative processes are promoted, functioning of internal organs is normalised and general condition is improved. Therefore, it ensues that antiparabiotic effect that is determined by replacement of strong or long acting monotonous stimulus of the nervous system by weak one makes the basis of therapeutic effect of procaine blockade. It should also be added that therapeutic effect of procaine blockade is in certain degree determined by pharmacological specificity and marked neurotropism of procaine. It is hydrolysed in tissues into para-amino benzoic acid (PABA) and diethyl aminoethanol. Products of its hydrolysis are long retained not only at the site of administration, but also in other parts of the body, influencing receptors, nerve conductors of somatic and vegetative nervous system, and nerve centres and modifying their functional state. Therefore, it is asserted that enervation effect on internal organs, vascular tone, endocrine glands and nerve centres of the somatic nervous system is modified by procaine blockade of individual ranges of somatic and especially vegetative nervous system. As a result, direct and reciprocal relationship of the periphery and nerve centres are normalized, neurohumoral regulation of impaired functions of the organism and its selected system is improved and recovery ensues.

The most pronounced therapeutic effect is seen in that part of somatic or vegetative nervous system, whose innervation segments have pathological focus and is exposed to procaine blockade. This is primarily determined by a peculiar multidimensional structure of sympathetic segment of the vegetative nervous system. The segmental relationship of prevertebral and paravertebral sympathetic ganglia with cerebrospinal segments and enervation relationship with peripheral and internal organs via postganglionic fibres that enter them together with blood vessels (Fig. 1). Thus, receiving preganglionic fibres from the first six thoracic segments, the cranial cervical sympathetic ganglion directs postganglionic sympathetic fibres to blood vessels that serve eyes, glands and other parts of the head, as well as to vessels of the pharynx, larynx and trachea. This is exactly why procaine blockade of the cranial sympathetic ganglion exerts immediate, primary effect on the vascular system of the head and other organs via post-ganglionic nerve fibres. Secondary effect that is mediated by subcortical centres and cerebral cortex due to impulses, coming from the blocked ganglion through preganglionic fibres and conduction tract of the spinal cord, occurs simultaneously. This secondary effect of the central origin influences the periphery by "all-in" principle, first, the site of affected organ, wherever it could be. It ensues, therefore, that, if there is a pathologic focus at area of the head, procaine blockade of cranial sympathetic ganglion has "double influence" on it: Primary (immediate) and secondary (mediated by nerve centres). Other sites of the body and pathologic foci that are away from the head accept intermediate, tropic and other effector impulses that equally affect function and tropism of all organs of the body during pathological process. The procaine blockade of prevertebtal and paravertebral sympathetic ganglia and plexuses exert double therapeutic effect (primary and secondary) on pathologic foci, located within the site of their enervation influence, and secondary effect on pathologic foci, outlying this site, and also on function of all organs and systems of the body.

The procaine blockade of medial (middle) cervical sympathetic ganglion will render via postganglionic fibres that innervate the vascular system of neck and forelimbs, a greater therapeutic effect in pathway of these parts of the body than blockade of cranial sympathetic ganglion. The blockade of stellate ganglion will, like blockade of the next three sympathetic ganglia and the sympathetic trunk, produce better therapeutic effect in pathology of forelimbs, withers and thoracic organs.

Types of procaine blockade: Depending on administration procaine solution into different sites of somatic and vegetative nervous system, the following types of procaine blockade are distinguished. Blockade of exteroceptors (skin, conjunctiva, nasal and oral mucosa) and of interoceptors delivering procaine solution into anatomical cavities (visceral receptors of abdominal and thoracic cavities, visceral receptors of synovial membranes of joints and tendon sheaths and intraosseous receptors).

Procaine blockade of extero and introceptors: Procaine blockade of extroceptor of the skin is done in internal organ diseases, neuritis, eczema and other cutaneous diseases. Intradermal procaine blockade of neck withers zone at the involved site is effective enough in pneumonia, pleuritis, neuritis of the neck and fore limbs, eczema of forelimbs, and in eczema of neck and withers blockade of contralateral side is effective. The neck-withers area is situated aside from the neck crest and the withers, beginning from the level of 2nd cervical vertebra and as far as top of the withers (spinous process of 5th thoracic vertebra). Its width is 7-10 cm in large animals and 2-3 cm in small animals. The punctures are spaced at interval of 1.5-2 cm. Warm procaine solution 0.25% (0.2 to 0.3 ml) is injected into each site.

In lumbosacral radiculitis, ischias, other neurites and eczema of the hind limb, skin receptors are blocked at area of the croup, beginning from the line which connects line as for as the level of the first caudal vertebra at the involved side (on contra lateral side if there is eczema of the croup area), aside from spinous processes of the sacrum; palm width in large animals 2-3 cm in small animals. The blockade is repeated at an internal of 2 to 3 days.

Procaine blockade of visceral receptors of the abdominal cavity is conducted in peritonitis, dyspepsia, gastroenteritis of calves in combination with sympathetic therapy. Weak solution of 0.25% procaine is intra-abdominally administered in a dose of 1 ml/kg of body weight in small animals, 0.5 ml/kg in large animals. Broad spectrum Penicillin and Streptomycin antibiotics are added in prescribed dose to procaine solution.

Technique (Large animals): Animals are restrained in the standing position. After observing asepsis perpendicular puncture of abdominal wall of calves and adult animals is done (at right side in cattle and left side in horses) at paralumbar fossa, in the middle distance between the last rib and loin, depth of puncture is 1 to 2 cm in calves and 3 to 4 cm in adult animals. The blockade is repeated at an interval of one day in peritonitis and 2 to 3 days in dyspepsia and gastroenteritis. Hussain and Kumar (1984) used procaine hydrochloride intraperitoneally in the management of abdominal surgery in buffaloes. The response to visceral pain after intraperitoneal administration of procaine was evaluated clinically and various abdominal surgical procedures viz., abomasotomy, spleenectomy, enterotomy were performed without any visceral response to pain after 0.5% procaine hydrochloride at the rate of 1 ml/kg in animals. Besides intraperitoneal administration, a linear infiltration of 5 to 7 ml of 2% local analgesia was given at the proposed site of incision. It produced a good analgesia and adequate relaxation of abdominal musculature that facilitated the successful completion of abdominal surgery. The blockade deflated the bowel that proved helpful in abdominal procedure.

Technique (Small animals): The intra-peritoneal injection was given in standing position through right paralumbar fossa in the middle of its upper third or fourth lumbar vertebrae. Skin and subcutaneous tissues are punctured with a blunt needle and it is inserted to a depth of a 20 to 30 mm, which varies according to age and development of musculature of the animal. The free entry of the solution with slight pressure indicated correct puncture. However, in dogs, visceral procaine blockade was induced after premedication of chlorpromazine by Hussain and Kumar (1984).

The administration of 0.5% procaine intraperitoneally with chlorpromazine premedication was evaluated clinically. Chlorpromazine hydrochloride was administered intramuscularly at the rate of 3 mg/kg body weight followed 10 minutes later by procaine hydrochloride 0.5% intraperitoneally at the rate of 1 ml/kg body weight. To complete surgical procedure the animal also received linear local infiltration of 2 to 3 ml of 2% local analgesia at the site of incision. Various abdominal surgical operations, viz., gastrotomy, enterotomy, spleenectomy, caecectomy, cystotomy, ovariohysterectomy were performed. The duration of surgery lasted for 90 minutes. It produced good anaesthesia and adequate relaxation of abdominal musculature facilitating successful completion of abdominal surgery. The intraperitoneal administration of 0.5% procaine with chlorpromazine premedication can be used successfully in canine surgery without any adverse effect on cardiovascular and respiratory system and on liver and kidney. Hussain and Kumar (1984) administered xylazine at the rate of 3 mg/kg body weight intramuscularly before intraperitoneal administration of 0.5% procaine hydrochloride in dogs. In order to desensitise the site of operation, the dogs are also given linear local infiltration of 2 to 3 ml of 2% local anaesthetic agent. The intraperitoneal injection is given on either side of the abdomen about 3 to 4 cm away from umbilicus in dogs. The analgesic effect of procaine hydrochloride 0.5% with premedication of xylazine produced good analgesia for 90 to 120 minutes in dogs. There was adequate relaxation of abdominal musculature that facilitated the successful completion of abdominal surgery. Intraperitoneal administration of 0.5% procaine hydrochloride with xylazine premedication might be used successfully in canine surgery.

Infraorbital procaine blockade in pathology of eye and adjoining structures:

Technique: The first line is drawn from lateral canthus of the eye parallel with ridge of the nose, the second one is perpendicularly made at the anterior edge of the first maxillary premolar. The site of intersection is infraorbital foramen in cattle and sheep. In horses a straight line parallel to the facial crest is drawn from internal canthus of the eye. Second line is drawn perpendicular to the first line beginning from the facial crest. About 1 to 2 cm from the intersection towards the nostril is the infraorbital foramen (Fig. 8). Procaine 0.5% is administered (horse and cattle: 40 to 60 ml, calf and sheep: 10 to 20 ml) and 30 to 40 ml & 10 to 15 ml are also given subcutaneously around the orbit. The blockade is repeated in 3 to 5 days.

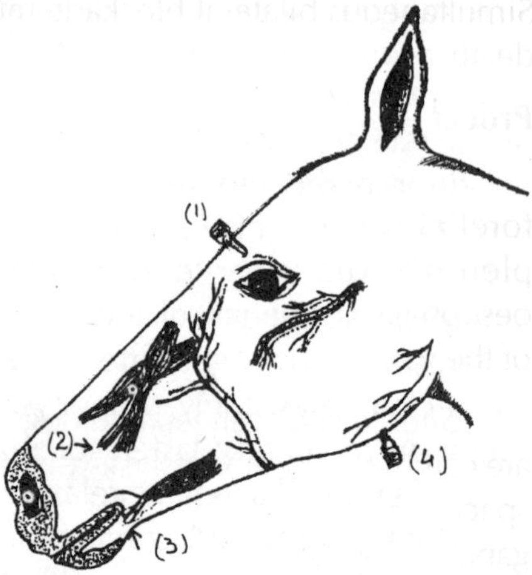

Fig. 8: Perineural injection of the sensory nerves in horse's head. Sites for insertion of the needle to block Supra orbital (1), Infra orbital (2), Mental (3) and Mandibular nerves (4)

Procaine blockade of medial cervical sympathetic ganglion, sympathetic trunk and vagus: In horses, cattle and other animals, these ganglia usually fuse with first two to three sympathetic ganglia and they together form the stellate ganglia, lying in the thoracic cavity nearby and behind the head of the first rib. The medial cervical sympathetic ganglion lies at the anterior edge of the first rib.

Technique: Large animals are restrained in the chute, the forelimb is drawn back, the head and neck are turned in contralateral direction. Transverse costal process of the 7th cervical vertebra is palpated above the jugular notch and in front of scapulo-humeral joint and vertical line is dropped from its anterior outline. Three to four cm receded downwards the line the site is located. Puncture is perpendicularly made to the skin as far as trachea. Warm procaine solution (50 to 60 ml) is injected slowly on right or left side. Slight resistance felt at administering the solution indicate proper position of the needle point.

Simultaneous bilateral blockade must never be done, because, death may ensue due to cardiac arrest.

Procaine blockade of stellate sympathetic ganglion:

Indications: Inflammatory processes at the area of the neck, forelimb, exudative bronchitis, lung oedema, pneumonia, pleuritis, diseases of heart and thoracic segment of the oesophagus. When blockade is properly done, thoracic segment of the vagus is not blocked.

Site: In cattle, sheep and dogs, stellate sympathetic ganglia are commonly located at the level of proximal 1/4 of first intercostal space, 2 to 3 cm below the head of the first rib. In horses, the ganglia have the same position of the right and are nearly protected by the second rib or are at the level of the second intercostal space of the left. In all animals it lies on lateral surface of long cervical muscle and is surrounded by loose fatty tissue and protected with pleura at the side of thoracic cavity.

Technique: Large animals are restrained in the chute, the forelimb of side is maximally drawn back, while the neck is turned to contralateral side. Small animals are restrained in the standing position or in lateral recumbence. The needle is inserted behind palpable tuberosity of the first rib and 2 to 3 cm below it. Warm 0.25% procaine solution is intradermally injected here. Thereafter the needle is advanced at a shallow angle backwards and inside until it strikes posterior edge of the first rib, the solution of the local analgesia is administered. The needle is displaced from the edge, till intercostal muscles are punctured and the needle is advanced until it strikes the body of the vertebra. As soon as the needle touches the body of the vertebra procaine solution is injected again at slow rate, resistance being felt. Going on with injection of provocaine, the needle is gradually withdrawn and, as soon as its point emerges at the surface of the muscle in the epipleural connective tissue space, resistance at the plunger until be considerably less, although still felt. This indicates proper position of the needle, without displacing the needle, the whole amount of procaine is gradually injected, 20 to 30 ml to large

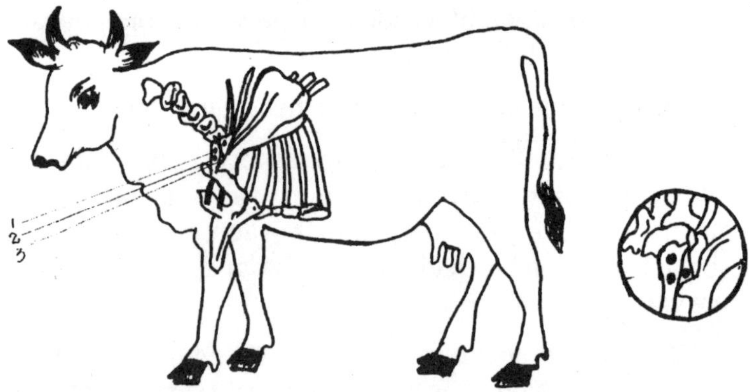

1. Head of the first rib
2. Site of inserting the needle until it strikes posterior edge of rib
3. First intercostal space

Fig. 9: Scheme of determination of the site of inserting the needle for procaine blockage of sympathetic stellate ganglion in cattle

animals, 5 to 10 ml to small animals. Free unrestricted administered of the solution indicates its entrance with the pleural cavity (Fig. 9).

Epipleural procaine blockade: It is of great practical significance. It is employed both therapeutically and for anaesthesia of abdominal organs. However, not only anaesthesia of internal organs is obtained, but their blood circulation is normalised. Blood pressure is stabilised, functional disorders of organs and systems are corrected, prelum abdominale is relaxed, post-operative peritonitis and atony of gastrointestinal tract, urinary bladder and uterus are prevented.

Indications: The block is indicated in diseases of lungs, cardiovascular system, acute and chronic ruminal atony, acute tympany, gastritis, enteritis, diseases of liver, spleen, kidneys and adrenal glands, dyspepsia in calves, delayed placental detachment, mastitis, inflammatory processes of penis and scrotum, eczemas, dermatitis, oedemas, tropic ulcers, long persistent wounds, especially those of thoracic and abdominal wall, back, croup and hind limbs. Acute serous, purulent, catarrhal, haemorrhage and fibrinous mastitis.

Technique: The method consists of administering 0.25 to 0.5% procaine solution in front of cruses of diaphragm into epipleural fatty tissue, surrounding the adjoining sympathetic trunk and celiac nerves. The technique of blockade is principally the same in all species.

Horses and cattle are restrained in a chute. Operative site is performed on both sides at the base of the last rib. Anterior edge of the last rib is found with index finger of the right hand. The finger is advanced towards the spine as far as intermuscular notch that is located between the iliocostal muscle and the longest muscle of the back. The needle is inserted at the site of intersection of the mentioned notch with vertical line, drawn from anterior edge of the last rib. A fine needle is inserted into the site of puncture and 2 to 3 ml of 0.5% procaine are injected intradermally, subcutaneously and intramuscularly. Then 12 cm long needle is taken. It is directed to horizontal surface at an angle of 30° to 35° and with quick but strong stab the skin is pierced and the needle is advanced parallel to the edge of the last rib until it strikes the body of the vertebra (Fig.10).If blood does not ooze from the

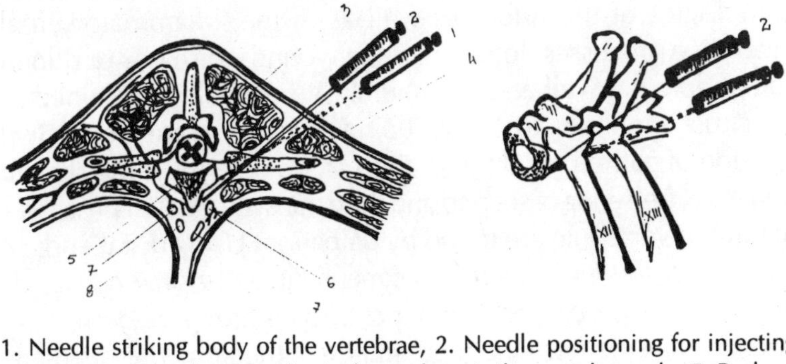

1. Needle striking body of the vertebrae, 2. Needle positioning for injecting solution , 3. Dorsal group of spinal muscles , 4. Ilio costal muscle, 5. Body of lumbar vertebrae, 6. Celiac nerve and sympathetic ganglion of adjoining trunk, 7. Bilateral veins, left and right, 8. Aorta

Fig. 10: Scheme of epipleural blockade of hypogastric nerves and sympathetic trunk

needle and air is not sucked by the thoracic cavity, the needle is fixed with the left hand, syringe with warm 0.25% or 0.5% procaine solution is adjusted to it. Pressing its plunger with the finger of the right hand, the needle and the syringe are deflected with the left hand 5° to 10° towards the sagital plane. As a result, free end of the needle somewhat departs from the vertebral body and the needle acquires posterior, parallel to ventrolateral surface of the vertebral body. Steadily pressing the plunger of the syringe, the needle is gently advanced until resistance at plunger is less and entrance of solution into epipleural loose fatty tissue is easier. To ascertain that position of the needle is proper, the syringe is separated. Emerging droplets of solution from the needle and its pulsation simultaneously with respiration are indicative of proper position. If the solution freely effuses from the syringe under plunger's weight then it pours out into the pleural cavity. In this case the needle should be carefully retracted several millimeters and pulsating droplets should be obtained. Procaine solution is administered in a dose of 0.5 ml/kg body weight. Total dose is divided in half and equal amounts are injected into right and left side. One blockade is sufficient for obtaining therapeutic effect in acute pathological processes. It is repeated in 5 to 7 days in subacute and chronic ones. Paravertebral and perineal procaine blockade of the udder are indicated in mastitis and other pathologies of the udder as well as in the inflammatory and ulcerative processes, long persisting wounds, diseases of skin of soft abdominal wall and perineum. The animal is restrained in the chute. Iliohypogastric and ilioinguinal nerves are blocked on the side of pathological focus (Fig.11). To determine the sites of puncture, free ends of second and third transverse costal processes of lumbar vertebrae are found by palpation. Using distal ends of these processes as references, segmental lines are drawn towards their spinous processes. The puncture sites are located on these lines 5 cm aside from the median line of the lion. The needle is perpendicularly inserted as deep as 6 to 8 cm until it strikes distal ends of 2nd and 3rd transverse costal processes, then displacing the needle somewhat backwards, it is inclined forward and deepened 0.5 to 0.75 cm and about 20 ml of warm 0.5% procaine

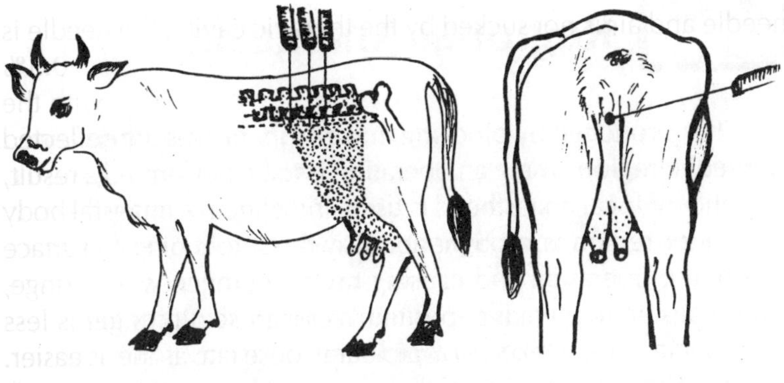

A B

Fig. 11: Scheme of procaine blockade in bovine mastitis
A = Paravertebral Blockade; B = Perineal procaine blockade

solution are administered into every site, changing position of the needle forward and backward. As both anterior portions of the udder are affected, the blockade is done at either side. If posterior portions are also involved, perineal nerves are blocked too. The operator puts an animal's tail left side. The operator raises lower vaginal commisure with the left hand and grasps ischiatic notch under it. The operator horizontally inserts the needle at this site as deep as 1.5 to 2 cm and directing its part to the right and to the left, injects 20 to 30 ml of 0.5% procaine solution.

10 Regional Analgesia

It is produced by blocking the sensory nerves innervating a particular region where an operation is to be performed. A small quantity of local anaesthetic is used and effective anaesthesia of the wider region is brought about without touching the actual site of the operation and causing no interference with healing. The anaesthetic agent is deposited in close viscinity of the nerves and special care is taken to avoid sheet of fascia, as the solutions do not diffuse through fascial sheets. However, this needs thorough knowledge of topographical anatomy of the nerves and the sites for injection. Success in regional anaesthesia is achieved with practice. Regional anaesthesia in large animals is practiced not only for surgery but also for diagnosis, prognosis and even for therapeutic reasons.

METHODS OF PRODUCING REGIONAL ANALGESIA

Paravertebral analgesia: Regional anaesthesia of the trunk in bovines is brought about by blocking the sensory conduction of spinal nerves as they emerge from the intervertebral foramina. This technique was introduced by Farquharson in 1940 and is used in bovine surgery for the operations of laparotomy and rumenotomy. During this regional anaesthesia the abdominal wall, including the peritoneum, is completely and uniformly desensitized. Muscular relaxation is produced and intra-abdominal pressure is decreased. The post-surgical convalescent period is shorter and of no consequence. The method is safe. The post-surgical convalescent period is shorter and there is saving of local analgesic solution. The area of the flank is innervated by the dorsal and ventral branches of thirteenth dorsal (T_{13}) and first and second lumbar (L_1 and L_2) nerves. The third lumbar nerve gives off a cutaneous branch that passes obliquely backwards in front of the ilium (Fig.12). The last dorsal foramen lies immediately caudal to the head of the last rib and on a level with the base of the transverse process of the first lumbar vertebra. The lumbar foramina are large and are situated between the bases of the transverse

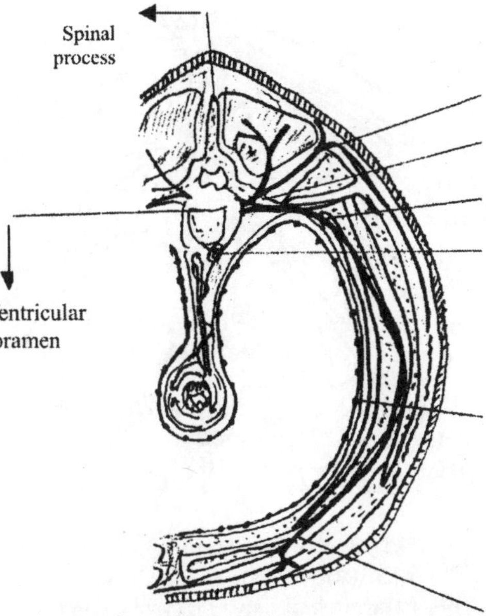

Fig. 12: Innervation of abdominal wall in cattle

processes and approximately on the same level. The spinal nerves, after emerging from the foramina, immediately divide into a smaller dorsal and a larger ventral branch. The former supplies chiefly the skin and muscles of the loins. The ventral branch passes obliquely ventrally and caudally between the muscles and innervates mainly to the skin, muscles and peritoneum of the flank. The ventral branch is also connected with the sympathetic system by a ramús communicans. Desensitization of the nerves at their point of emergence from the intervertebral foramina will provide anaesthesia of the whole depth of the flank wall and complete muscular relaxation. Due to the deep location of the nerves and lack of absolute precision for detection of landmark the paravertebral block cannot be induced with absolute certainty. It is probable that blocking of dorsal branch is automatic if the larger, ventral branch is effectively contacted and desensitization of the flank is complete. The number of nerves to be blocked will depend on the site and extent of the incision to be made (Fig.13). For rumenotomy operation, the incision is parallel with and about 7 cm behind last rib. Blocking of thirteenth thoracic and the first lumbar nerve is adequate, whereas for caesarean section by flank incision it is necessary to inject the first, second and third lumbar nerves.

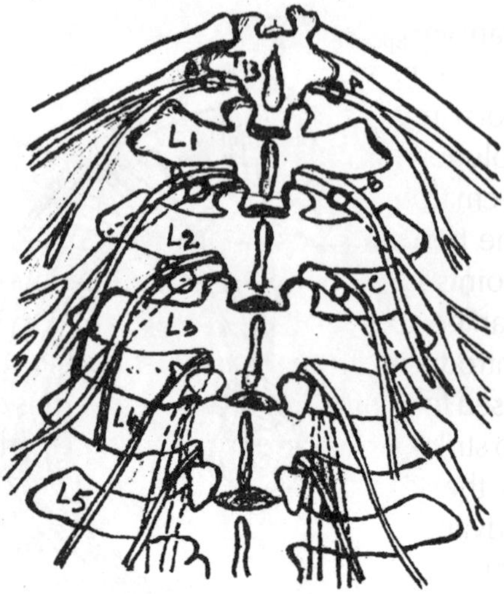

Fig. 13: Needle placement for blockade of T13 (A), L1(B) & L2(C) nerves for Paravertebral nerve block of cattle.

Technique: The site is located by palpating the last rib with the index finger. The head of the rib can be felt about 5 cm lateral to the mid-line. This marks the site for the injection of the thirteenth thoracic nerve. To determine the sites for the lumbar nerves, a transverse line is drawn immediately behind the spinous process of the particular vertebra and the needle is inserted at a point on this line 5 cm from the mid-line. The nerve lies at a depth of about 5 cm. An insensitive skin weal is first produced, using a short and comparatively fine needle (20 gauge, 3 cm long) and injecting about 3 ml of solution. These weals are raised in line with most obvious parts of the transverse processes of the second, third and fourth lumbar vertebrae, about 5 cm from the midline of the body. Since the location of the transverse process of the first lumbar vertebra is difficult so that in most cases the site for infiltration around the thirteenth thoracic nerve is formed by simple measurement. The distance between the skin weals over the second and third lumbar transverse processes is measured and another skin weal is produced at a distance equal to this in front of the anterior weal. This marks the site where the needle is to be introduced to strike the anterior border of the first lumbar transverse process. A stout needle (7 cm long, 3 mm bore) is inserted through each skin weal and the underlying longissimus dorsi muscle is infiltrated with 2 to 3 ml of local anaesthetic solution through these needles as they are advanced to a depth of 4 cm from the skin surface. The needles used for injections around the nerves (10 cm long, 2 mm bore) should have 'short bevel' points so that penetration of the tough intertransverse ligament can be appreciated as the needle is advanced. These needles are introduced through the holes made in the skin by the stout needles used for infiltration of the longissimus dorsi muscle, and advanced to strike the anterior border of the vertebral process. Each needle is then redirected forwards over the edge of the process and advanced until it is felt to penetrate the intertransverse ligament. Injection of 15 ml of 2% lignocaine Hcl with 1:40,000,00 adrenaline is made immediately below the ligament and a further 5 ml of this solution is injected as the needle is withdrawn, to just above the ligament. It is important to ensure that the needle shall be vertical when contact is first made with the anterior border of the processes. Successful infiltration of the nerves is indicated by the development of a belt of hyperaemia, which causes an appreciable rise in the skin temperature. Full anaesthesia develops in about 10 minutes and persists for about 90 minutes. A lateral curvature of the spine towards the anaesthetized side will be noted. Failure to block the dorsal branches of the nerves is evidenced by skin sensitivity dorsal to the mid-fossa region. Failure to block the ventral branches is evidenced by skin sensitivity ventral to the mid-fossa region. This technique was developed which has proved to be satisfactory even in the hands of inexperienced students.

In sheep and goats, a similar technique to that of cattle is satisfactory. The injection site is 3 cm from the mid-line. Palpation of the transverse processes of the lumbar vertebra presents no difficulty, and because the nerves lie nearer to the skin surface the injection can be made with greater precision than in cattle. Full analgesia develops in 5 minutes and persists for 60 minutes.

In case of dogs, paravertebral block of the last three thoracic and first four lumbar nerves affords a useful, safe method of producing relaxation of the abdominal muscles. Used in conjunction with light general anaesthesia it produces excellent operating conditions for the surgeon working within the abdomen. It is necessary to block seven nerves on each side of the body and, clearly, this is a time-consuming procedure. However, when combined with light general anaesthesia, it is a technique which is very useful under conditions of general practice, since it produces operating conditions equal to those obtained by the use of muscle relaxants, yet it does not necessitate the IPPV of the lungs which must be employed when relaxants are used.

Pudic (internal pudendal) nerve block: This nerve is derived from the ventral branches of the spinal nerves S_3 and S_4 and occasionally S2 and passes caudoventral on the medial surface of the sacrosciatic ligament. It receives an anastomosing branch from the sciatic nerve at the lesser sciatic foramen.

The pudendal nerve gives off a proximal and a distal cutaneous branch to the caudal femoral region. It also gives branches to the skin and muscles of the vulva (labia) of the cow or the skin and muscle derivatives of the embryonic cloacal sphincter of the bull, and a superficial perineal or a mammary branch to the upper caudal part of scrotum. It terminates as the nervus clitoridis in the female and the nervus dorsalis penis in the bull. The latter innervates the retractor penis muscle, the glans penis region and part of the prepuce. The hemorrhoidal nerve (S_1 and S_2) supplies the skin and muscles (medial and lateral coccygeal) of the anus and perineum.

This nerve block is indicated for examination, treatment and surgery of the penis. Caudal epidural anaesthesia is preferable for surgery of the vulvar and perineal regions. The technique was developed by Larson in 1953 who claimed the following main advantages of the internal pudendal nerve block:

i) The technique consistently results in anaesthesia of the penis and relaxation of the retractor penis muscle.

ii) Special stocks are not required, but if used the bull can be removed from them immediately after the operation is completed because full use of the pelvic limbs is retained.

iii) A sedative is not necessary when protracting or manipulating the penis.

iv) The bull can be treated in the standing position. Casting has been frequent with epidural method.

Technique: The technique comprises appropriate skin preparation. Anaesthetic is injected subcutaneously besides the anus at the deepest point of the ischiorectal fossa, through a 1 to 2 cm, 13 or 14 gauge needle inserted through the skin. With the hand in the rectum, a 12 to 25 cm, 18 gauge needle is passed through the larger sciatic foramen. The needle is guided to the pudendal and hemorrhoidal nerves, and 25 ml of 2% lignocaine is injected at the sites indicated (Fig.14).The contralateral pudendal and hemorrhoidal nerves are blocked similarly.

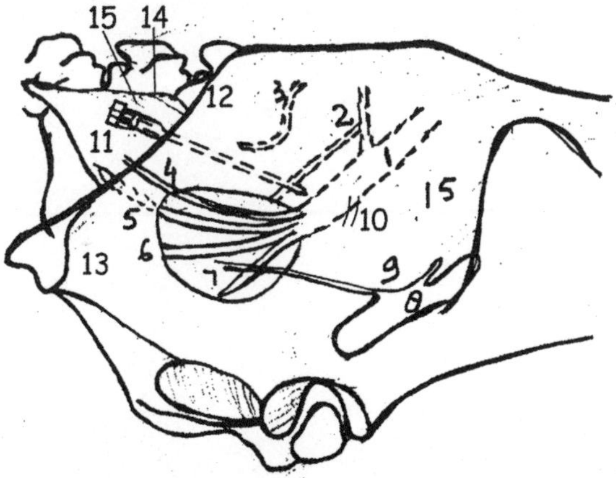

1. Pudic Nerve 2. Middle haemorrhoidal nerve 3. Caudal haemorrhoidal nerve 4,5. Proximal and distal cutaneous branches of pudic nerve, 6. Deep perineal nerve, 7. Dorsal nerve of pelvis, 8. Sciatic nerve, 9. Branch connecting sciatic nerve with branch of pudic nerve (7), 10. Pelvis nerve, 11. Coccygeus muscle, 12. Sacrosciatic ligament, 13. Tuber ischii, 14. First coccygeal vertebrae, 15. Needle in position.

Fig. 14: Needle placement for pudic nerve block in the bull with lateral view of dissection of pelvis

The pudendal nerve is located by palpation in the following manner: (1) Locate the lesser sciatic notch and foramen, (2) locate the internal iliac (pudendal) artery at the cranial angle of this notch, (3) move the hand craniad and locate the superior ischiatic spine, (4) palpate the pudendal nerve just caudodorsad to the internal iliac artery, (5) after injection of anaesthetic over the pudendal nerve, additional anaesthetic is injected caudodorsad to anaesthetize the hemorrhoidal nerves.

The pudendal nerve may also be blocked in sheep using digital palpation of the lesser sacrosciatic foramen as a guide.

11 Regional Anaesthesia Techniques

HEAD REGION:

Infraorbital nerve block: The infraorbital nerve emerges on the face through the infraorbital foramen, where it is partly covered by the levator nasolabialis muscle. It is a sensory nerve. During its course it supplies sensory fibers to the upper lip and cheek, the nostrils and lower parts of the face. Nerve is blocked (i) at the point of its emergence from the infraorbital foramen, where it will desensitize the skin of the upper lip, nostril and face on that side up to the level of the foramen. (ii) within the canal through infraorbital foramen to desensitize the first and second premolars, the canine and incisor teeth with their alveoli and gum, and the skin as high as the level of the inner canthus of the eye. (iii) within the pterygopalatine fossa at the point the nerve enters the maxillary foramen, in which case, besides the structures outlined in (i) and (ii), the cheek teeth three to six will be desensitized.

Indications: Surgical management of conditions of upper lip and nostrils, (i.e., suturing of wounds, removal of polyps), extraction of canine or incisor teeth and trephining of facial sinuses.

Technique: The infraorbital nerve of the horse may be blocked at three sites: (i) Blockade at the infraorbital foramen. The foramen in the horse lies approximately 1 to 2 cm. superior to the midpoint of an imaginary line between the anterior extremity of the facial crest and the nasomaxillary notch. The lip of the foramen can usually be palpated beneath the levator nasolabialis muscle. In cattle and buffalo the foramen is felt as a depression on a line connecting the medial canthus and the nostril. A 20 gauge 5 cm. needle is inserted into the lip of the foramen and about 10 ml. of 2% lignocaine or other local anaesthetic is injected, (ii) To block the nerve in the infraorbital canal a 20 gauge 5 cm. needle is inserted 2 to 3 cm. anterior to the foramen and 5 to 10 ml. of local anaesthetic agent is injected to desensitize the canine and incisor teeth with associated alveoli and gum and the skin below the medial canthus of eye. (iii) Before entering into the infraorbital canal the nerve is called maxillary nerve. The nerve can be blocked at this site when the needle is inserted 2 to 3 cm. below the lateral canthus of the eye (just ventral to the facial crest) in a medial slightly dorsoanterior direction. The needle is passed 6-8 cm deep along the posterior surface of the maxillary tuberosity to the maxillary foramen. Care is to be taken to avoid the puncture of maxillary artery (Fig.8 & 15).

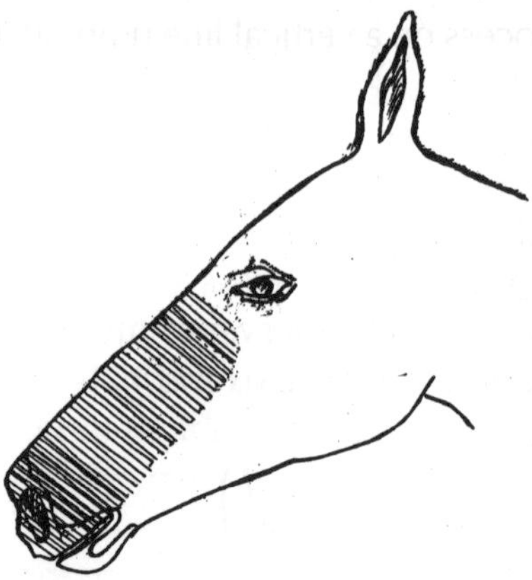

Fig. 15: Area of skin desensitized after blocking the infra-arbitral nerve within the canal (Horizontal lines)

An insensitive skin wheel, before actual block, is an advantage. Loss of sensation should follow in 15 - 20 minutes and last a further 30 - 40 minutes if the solution injected contains a vasoconstrictor.

Supraorbital (frontal) nerve block: Supraorbital nerve is a branch of the ophthalmic nerve and emerges through the supraorbital foramen. The nerve continues across the periorbita through the frontal (supraorbital) foramen, and innervates the middle portion of the upper lid and the temporal skin and some part of the skin of the forehead. Nerve block is performed in the horse and cattle.

Indications: Operations above the upper eyelids, suturing of skin wounds in the forehead region, and trephining of the frontal sinus.

Technique: The foramen is located as a small pit-like depression midway between the two borders of supraorbital process on a vertical line running upwards from the medial angle of the eye. The skin is prepared and an insensitive wheel produced. The needle is inserted 0.5 to 1.0 cm. deep. About 5 ml. (2%) lignocaine HCl is injected. In cattle needle is inserted a little above the medial canthus and directed laterally along the supraorbital process towards the temporal region. During withdrawal a transverse injection of 5 to 10 ml. (2%) lignocaine HCl is made (Fig.16 and 17).

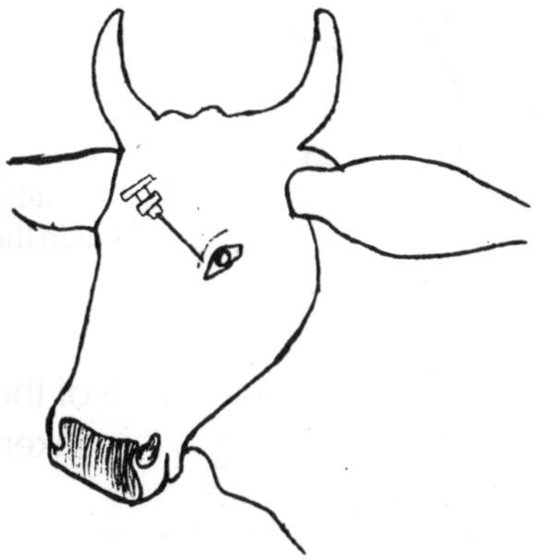

Fig. 16: Needle placement for supra-arbitral nerve block in cattle

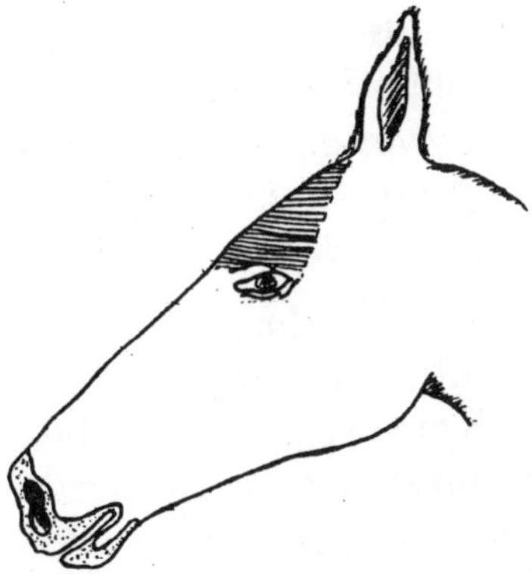

Fig. 17: Area of skin desensitized after blocking supra-arbitral nerves (Horizontal lines)

Maxillary nerve block: The block is performed in horse, cattle, dog and cat. To avoid the danger involved in blocking the nerve within the pterygopalatine fossa (as it may result in the damage to buccal vein and other vessels) it was recommended that the maxillary nerve be blocked at its exit from the round foramen. The block desensitizes upper jaw with its teeth and gum, lower half of nasal cavity, lower eyelid and skin over the muzzle and upper lip.

Indications: Surgical management of conditions of the upper lip, nose and upper jaw.

Technique: The site is located on the aboral surface of zygomatic process of the frontal bone, close to the external frontal crest, and above 1 cm. anterior to the point where the temporalis muscle runs deeply. This site is a hand's breadth medial to the mandibular joint. A needle about 12 cm. long is inserted here at right angle to the frontal bone and inclined 20^0 medially to a depth about one and a half times the diameter of the orbit. This distance should first be measured and needle marked accordingly, 10 ml. of 2% lignocaine is administered here in horse or cattle. To avoid damage to any vessel, needle with a blunted point is recommended.

A 2 inch long, 18 gauge needle is inserted in line with the eye just below the zygomatic arch and directed towards the pterygopalatine fossa. Two to 4 ml. of 2% local anaesthetic is deposited at this site in dog and cat (Fig.18).

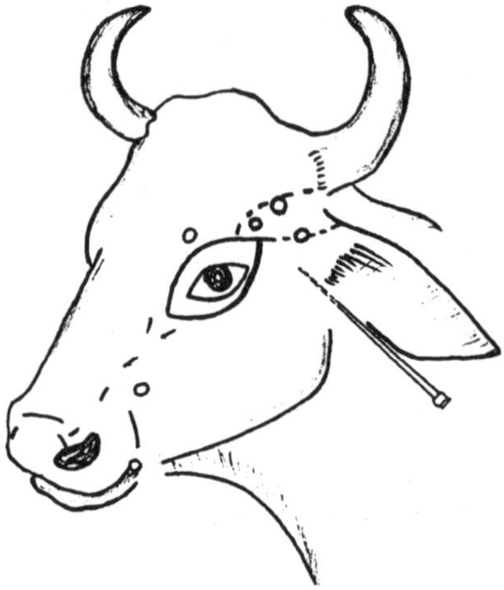

Fig. 18: Needle placement for maxillary nerve block in ox

Auriculopalpebral nerve block

The auriculopalpebral nerve comes from the facial branch of trigeminal nerve at the posterior border of the vertical ramus. It passes up in the parotid gland and divides into the anterior auricular and temporal branches. The former supplies branches to the muscles of the anterior auricular group while the latter supplies the orbicularis oculi and the corrugator muscles.

The auriculopalpebral nerve innervates orbicularis oculi muscle with motor fibbers. It continues to the inside of orbit and ramifies in several branches to the circular muscles of eye. In cattle the nerve trunk runs immediately over the facial crest past and below the eye, and gives off its branches on the way, whereas in the dog the nerve before reaching the orbit divides into two branches that continue medially and laterally to the eye. Blocking this nerve prevents voluntary closure of the eyelid but does not in any way desensitize them (akinesia).

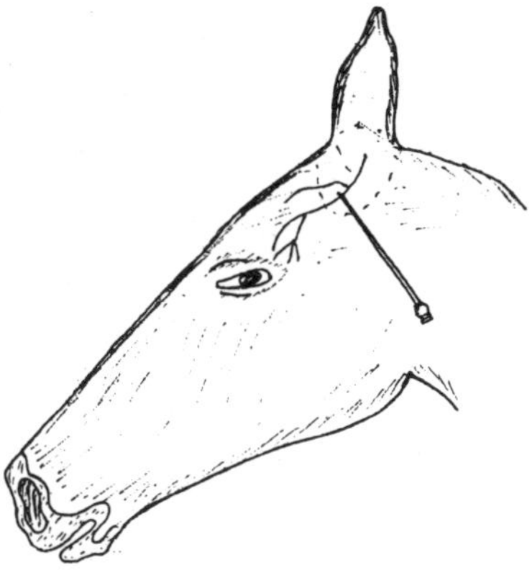

Fig. 19: Needle placement for auriculo palpebral nerve block in horse

Indications: In conjunction with topical analgesia of the conjunctiva it is most useful for examination of the eyeball, to relieve the spasms of the eyelids following an eye injury, surgical conditions of the eyelids and eyeball in conjunction with the retrobulbar nerve block. It is of particular value in preventing squeezing of the eyeball after intraocular operation.

Technique: In horse the site is 3 cm. below the highest point of the dorsal border of the zygomatic arch. The needle is inserted obliquely and dorsally to contact bone and is pushed along the bone until the point almost reaches the border of the zygomatic arch. Five milliliters of 2% anaesthetic solution is administered subfascially. In cattle, the needle is inserted directly to the aboral end of the zygomatic arch, and once in contact with bone, is pushed forward until its point lies at the dorsal border of the zygomatic arch. Ten to fifteen milliliters of 2% lignocaine is administered subfascially. In dog the needle is directed towards the middle of forehead, as it is inserted subfascially over the posterior third of the zygomatic arch, directly

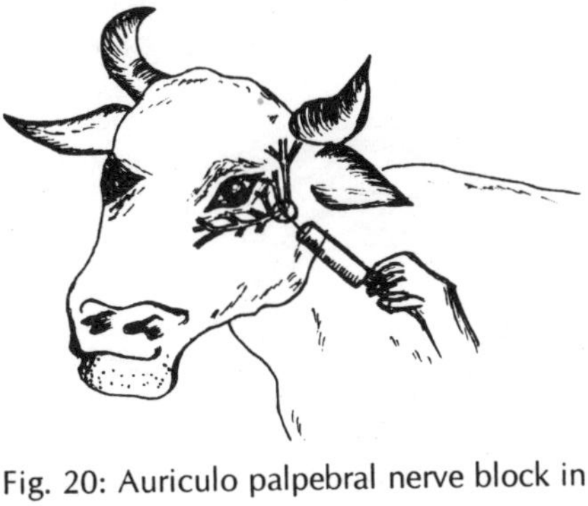

Fig. 20: Auriculo palpebral nerve block in Ox

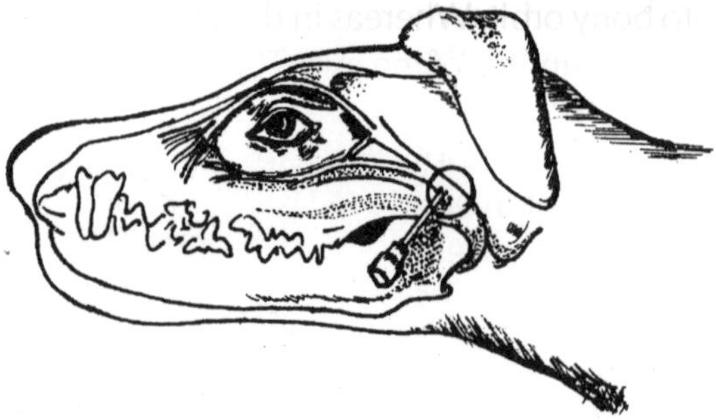

Fig. 21: Auriculo palpebral nerve block in Dog

above its dorsal border, one ml. of 2% local anaesthetic solution is injected (Fig. 19, 20 and 21).

Retrobulbar nerve block: This block is performed in horse, cattle and dog.

Indications: Surgical management of conditions of eyeball and membrane nictitans.

Technique: In horse retrobulbar injection is successfully used to anaesthetize the eyeball. To use this method the eyelids are anaesthetized with local infiltration. A 10 cm. long, 20 gauge needle is inserted 2 cm. behind the middle of the supraorbital process and directed towards the last upper premolar tooth on opposite side. Twenty to 30 ml. of 2% lignocaine Hcl is deposited after the needle has penetrated the orbit. Similar results are claimed by directing the needle from the medial or lateral margins of the orbit. In cattle retrobulbar infiltration is made in the same manner as outlined in horse. It is possible to enter the optic foramen from this approach, so the needle should not be inserted too far

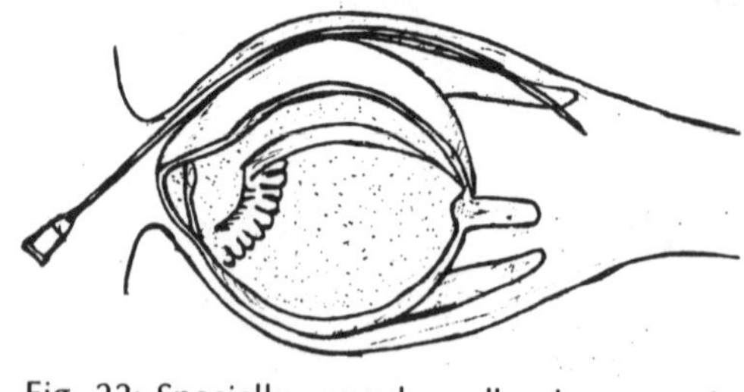

Fig. 22: Specially curved needle placement for producing retrobulbar anaesthesia

posteriorly into bony orbit. Whereas in dog, the needle is inserted through the lateral canthus of the eye. Three to 5 ml. of 2% local anaesthetic solution is injected to block the nerve. Use of specifically curved needles for retrobulbar anaesthesia to reduce the risk of complications has been recommended (Fig. 22, 23 and 24).

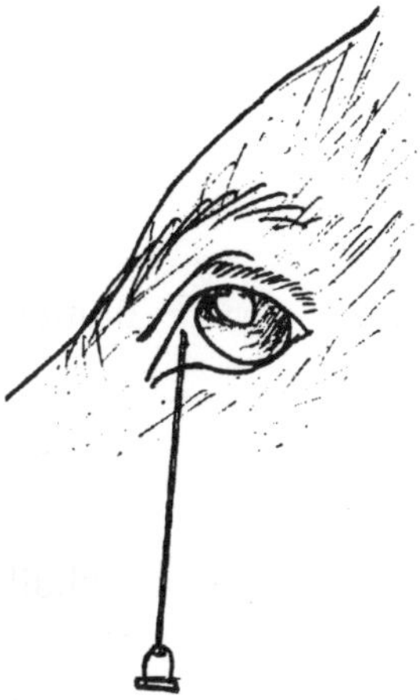

Fig. 23: Retrobulbar needle placement through the medial canthus

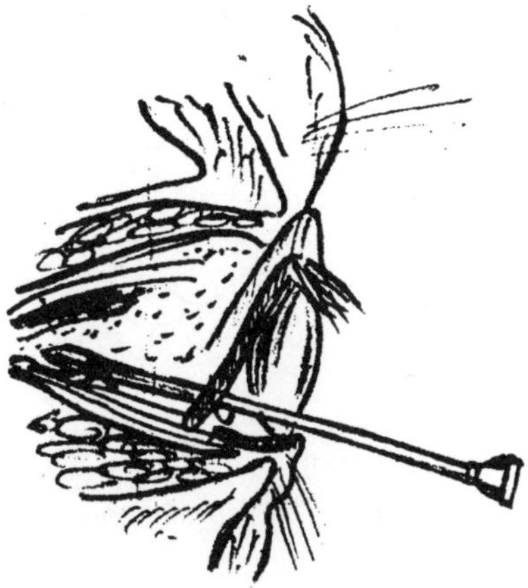

Fig. 24: Needle placement for retrobulbar nerve block to the orbital apex in cattle

Peterson's orbital nerve block: The block is commonly performed in cattle.

Indications: Surgical management of conditions of eye ball, eyelid and horns.

Technique: The orbital nerve block is performed to anaesthetize the third, fourth, sixth, ophthalmic and maxillary parts of fifth cranial nerves emerging from the foramen orbitorotundum. In cattle a 10 cm long curved 20 gauge needle is inserted in the caudal notch formed by the supraorbital process and zygomatic arch, passed craniomedial to the coronoid just rostral to the foramen orbitorotundum at a depth of about 8 - 10 cm from the skin. By moving the needle the boundary of the foramen is ascertained and 15 ml of 2% local anaesthetic solution is deposited into the periorbital cone in a ring like fashion which will desensitize the eyeball and horn simultaneously (Fig. 25).

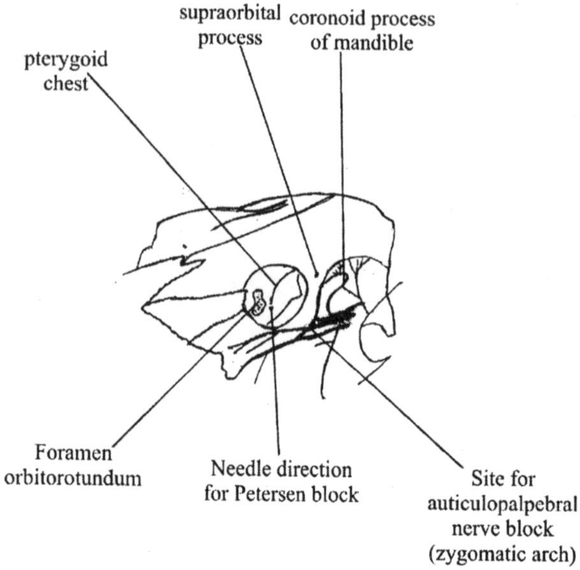

Fig. 25: Schematic drawing of the Peterson nerve block in cattle

Adverse effects of the Peterson and retrobulbar blocks result from penetration of blood vessels to produce orbital haemorrhage, direct pressure on the eyeball, damage to the optic nerve and injection of the optic nerve meninges, but clearly most are unimportant when the blocks are used for other purposes. Care must be taken to ensure that the corneal surface does not become dry because of loss of tear formation for several hours.

Cornual nerve block in cattle: This method was developed by Emmerson for cattle and by Vitums (1954) for goats in USA. The horns of cattle are supplied with sensory fibers through the cornual nerve, which is a branch of the lacrimal, one of the three branches of the ophthalmic nerve. The cornual nerve passes through periorbital tissue dorsally and then runs along lateral border of the frontal crest roofing temporal fossa at the base of the horn.

Indications: Dehorning in cattle and goats, occasional surgical interference in the same region.

Technique: The needle is inserted midway between the base of the horn and the lateral canthus of the eye. The site is located by palpating the frontal crest where the corneal nerve passes just below the crest subcutaneously, 10 ml of 2% lignocaine HCl solution is deposited around the nerve. In old cows and bulls, caudal aspect of horn skin may be supplied from the first cervical nerve, thereby requiring the infiltration of anaesthetic just posterior to the base of the horn.

In goats the nerve supply to the horn is from cornual branches of the lacrimal and the infratrochlear nerves. The cornual branches of the lacrimal nerve are blocked by inserting the needle just caudal to the beginning of the supraorbital process. To block cornual branch of infratrochlear nerve the site of injection is at the dorsomedial margin of the orbit above the eye. About 2 to 3 ml of 2% local anaesthetic solution should be injected at each site (Fig. 26 and 27).

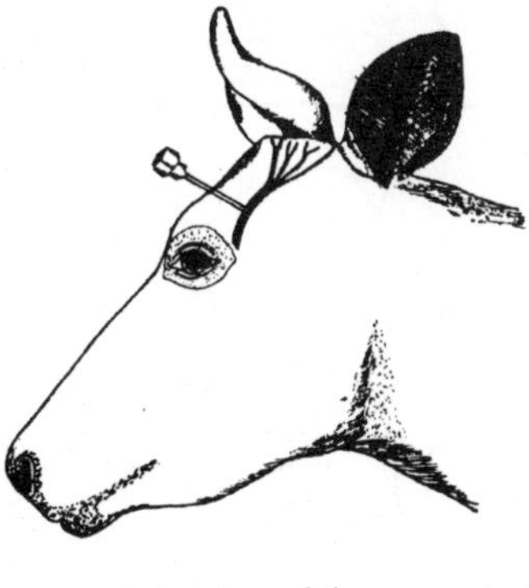

Fig. 26: Injection of the nerve to the horn core in the Ox

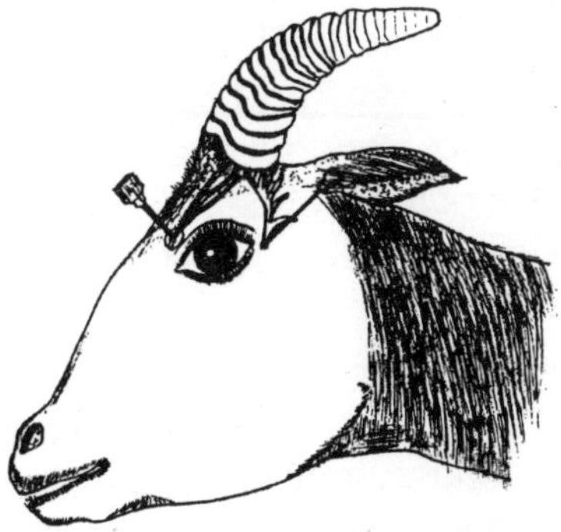

Fig. 27: Nerve block for dishorning of Goats

Lingual nerve block: The sensory nerve supply to tongue is from the lingual nerve which consists of lingual branch of fifth, the chorda tympani of the seventh and the lingual branch of the ninth cranial nerves. The hypoglossal nerve is the motor nerve to the tongue. For complete anaesthesia of the tongue both these nerves should be blocked. This type of anaesthesia is useful for general interference on the tongue anterior to the vallate papillae. Injection may be made from the mouth cavity or the intermaxillary space.

Indications: Surgical management of any condition of the tongue e.g., removal of foreign bodies, management of lacerations, cuts and ranula, immobilization of the tongue.

Technique: After securing the head of the animal, the mouth is opened with the help of Varnell's mouth gag. The tongue is held at the base and is withdrawn. To block the lingual nerve, a 15 cm long, 16 gauge needle is passed along the medial surface of fourth or fifth lower cheek tooth and introduced approximately 1.5 cm caudoventrally through the connective tissue. Ten milliliter of 2% local anaesthetic solution is injected at the site while withdrawing the needle.

To block the hypoglossal nerve, the needle is introduced in the longitudinal groove between bellies of the styloglossus and hyoglossus muscles caudoventrally at the base of the tongue. The needle is steadily introduced into the tongue as far posterior as possible and maneuvered to a depth of 1.5 to 2 cm intramuscularly. Ten milliliters of anaesthetic is injected at the site. Identical procedure is repeated on the opposite side (Fig. 28).

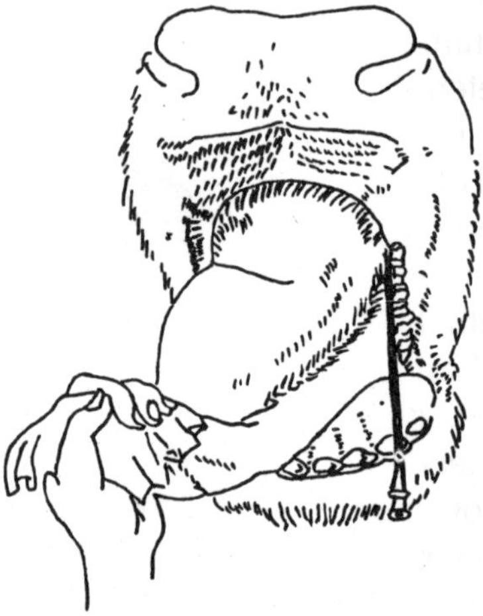

Fig. 28: Needle placement for lingual nerve block

Mandibuloalveolar nerve block: The inferior maxillary division of the trifacial or trigeminal nerve leaves the cranial cavity through the foramen ovale, runs downwards and forwards between the two pterygoid muscles, enters the mandibular foramen, passes along the mandibular canal, passes out this canal through the mental foramen, and finally breaks off into a number of labial (inferior) filaments while passing along the mandibular canal, gives off inferior dental and alveolar branches to the lower cheek teeth, gums and the alveolar periosteum. The terminal mental filaments supply the lower lip.

Indications: Management of surgical conditions of molar teeth and incisors and the body of the mandible in the lower jaw, suturing of the wounds of the lower lip.

Technique: Following two procedures can be used: (a) Facial approach: This approach is usually followed in large animals. The needle is inserted from the lower angle of the jaw along the medial surface of the ramus of the mandible at a point where a line along the masticatory surface of the mandibular cheek teeth is crossed by a perpendicular line through the lateral canthus of the eye. At the intersection of these two lines lies the mandibular foramen. The length of the needle may be chosen by first determining the distance from the point of insertion to the point of intersection of the two lines mentioned above. Then 15 to 20 ml of 2% local anaesthetic solution is injected at the site. (b) Oral approach: This approach is preferred for dog and cat. The needle is inserted medial and parallel to the long axis of the sixth molar with the point inclined towards the mandible. Then 2 to 4 ml of 2% anaesthetic solution is injected in the tissue around the nerve (Fig. 29). The technique is difficult and uncertain, for the nerve enters the canal high up in the medial aspect of vertical ramus. Most surgeons today prefer to carry out all dental surgery under general anaesthesia and this block will only be used when, for some reasons, general anaesthesia is unpracticable.

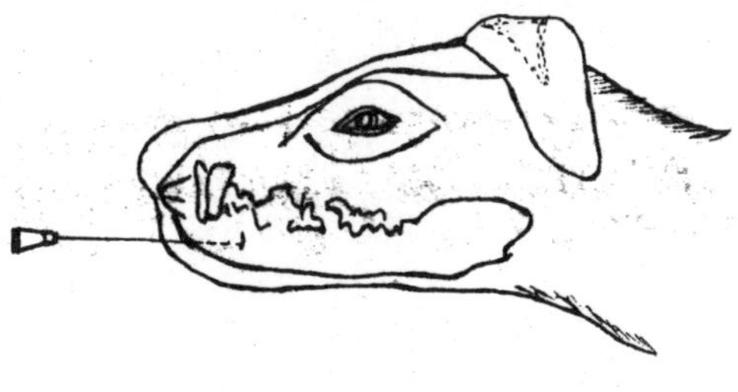

Fig. 29: Mandibuloalveolar nerve block in Dog

Mental nerve block: This block is performed in horse, cattle, dog and cat to anaesthetize the dental nerves of lower jaw in the mandibular canal and at the mental foramen.

Indications: Suturing of wounds of lower lip, wiring operations around the lower teeth and the body of the mandible.

Technique: The mental foramen is situated on the lateral aspect of the ramus in the middle of the interdental space in horse, or just behind fourth incisor in cow, or below the first molar in the dog and cat. The mental nerve is blocked by injecting a local anaesthetic solution into the canal (10 - 15 ml in horse and cattle and 1 - 2 ml in dog and cat). The mental foramen is palpated by holding the lower jaw just below the angle of the lips and with the tight grip the fingers are pushed upwards where the foramen is felt as a shallow depth in the bone. A 20 gauge, 3 to 4 cm long needle is adequate to deposit the anaesthetic solution at the foramen or up into the canal (Fig. 8 & 30).

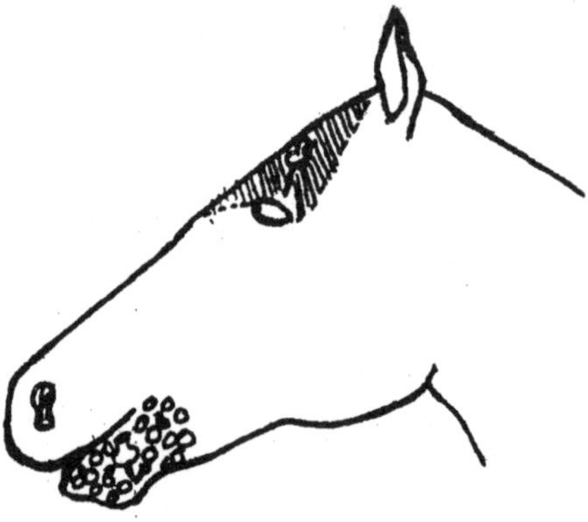

Fig. 30: Area of skin desensitization after blocking the mental nerve (spotted)

12 Regional Anaesthetic Blocks of the Fore Limb

The purpose for regional anaesthetic blocks for limbs is mainly to determine the specific area causing lameness, and to provide anaesthesia for surgical procedures.

The sensory innervation of the fore limb below the elbow is from the median and ulnar nerves and the musculocutaneous nerve. To obtain complete anaesthesia of the limb from carpus down, anaesthesia of the median nerve must therefore be combined with that of ulnar and the musculocutaneous nerves simultaneously.

MEDIAN NERVE (horse): The nerve is readily palpated 5 cm distal to the elbow joint on the medial aspect of the limb immediately behind the posterior border of the radius and in front of the muscular belly of the internal flexor of the metacarpus, deep to the caudal superficial pectoral muscle and the deep fascia.

Technique: With the animal standing, the operator stops slightly behind the opposite forelimb. The posterior border of the radius where it meets the lower edge of the caudal superficial pectoral muscle is located. The point for insertion of the needle is immediately above the finger. A suitable needle is directed upwards and inwards at an angle of 20 degree to the vertical to ensure penetration of the pectoral muscle and fascia. Five to 10 ml. of local anaesthetic solution is injected. To facilitate insertion of the needle to the proper depth it is best first to induce an insensitive skin weal. The surface area desensitized with median nerve block is little more than obtained with medial high palmar block. It takes 10 minutes before the area is desensitized. The chief indication for the block is operation for median neurectomy. The area desensitized in the fore limb is below the carpus.

Ulnar (horse): It is blocked at the centre of the posterior aspect of the limb, one hand's breadth above the carpal joint, in the groove between the tendons of the middle and external flexors of the metacarpus, and beneath the deep fascia, at a depth of 1 to 2 cm.

Musculocutaneous (horse): The internal aspect of the limb where the nerve lies on the surface of the radius, half-way between the elbow and carpus, immediately adjacent to the cephalic vein the musculocutaneous nerve is blocked.

Palmar/ Plantar nerve block: In horses it is the most common form of perineural block employed in veterinary practice. According to the site at which injection is made it is classified as high plantar, low plantar and subcarpal plantar block. High plantar block is the most important.

The palmar (metacarpal) nerves are those which confer sensibility to the digit. The internal (medial) palmar nerve of the forelimb is one of the terminal branches of the median nerve. It begins above the carpus, and at about the middle of the metacarpus it gives off a considerable branch, which winds obliquely behind the flexor tendons, to join the external palmar nerve above the button of the splint (4th metacarpal) bone. At the level of the proximal sesamoid bones the trunk of the nerve divides into three digital branches, which are distinguished as dorsal, middle and palmar. The palmar is the largest. The middle is the smallest and most irregular, and all the three branches are in close relationship with digital vessels. The dorsal branch descends and distributes cutaneous branches to the front of the digit, and terminates in the coronary cushion. The middle branch, which is union of several smaller branches terminates in the sensitive laminae and the coronary cushion. The palmar branch supplies the hoof to the ospedis and sensitive laminae.

The lateral palmar nerve of the forelimb is formed by the fusion of the termination of the ulnar nerve with one of the terminal branches of the median nerve at the upper border of accessory carpal bone. Behind the carpus the nerve inclines downwards and outwards, in the texture of the annular ligament that completes the tarsal sheath. In the metacarpal region it lies on the outside of the limb. At the level of the sesasmoid bones it divides into three digital branches exactly similar to those of the medial palmar nerve.

In the hind limb plantar nerves result from the bifurcation of the posterior tibial nerve when it gains the back of tarsus. A little below the middle of the metatarsus the medial nerve detaches a considerable branch that winds obliquely behind the flexor tendons joins the lateral planter nerve at the level of the button of the 4th metatarsal. At the fetlock each nerve, coming into relation with the digital vessels, resolves itself into three branches for supply of the digit. In the pastern region the disposition of the nerve and vessels is the same as in the forelimb. The nerve supply of the digit of the ox is much more complex than in the horse and regional analgesia is more difficult to produce. The skin below the carpus and tarsus is tense and the subcutaneous tissue is very fibrous, so that precise location of nerves is not easy. Many workers consider that simple ring block, in which a transverse plane through the whole extremity is infiltrated, is the most reliable way of producing regional analgesia of the digit. However, block of the individual nerves is more elegant.

High palmar/plantar injection: The site lies 5 - 7 cm. above the fetlock joint. The site is bounded anteriorly by suspensory ligament and posteriorly by deep digital flexor tendon and the depression is located. This groove lodges the vein, artery and the nerve, in the order of from before backwards. The nerve lies immediately to the anterior of the deep digital flexor tendon. A needle (1.5 cm, 19 gauge) is selected, the site is clipped and cleansed, and a twitch is applied to the animal. The operator stoops, down, facing the lateral aspect of the limb, and with a single thrust insert the needle at an angle of 15 degrees with the vertical, to its full extent. Since the skin and fascia are tense, in standing animal, it is easy to penetrate the skin and the subsequent injection is in direct contact with the nerve, just above the division of the nerve. It is ensured that the needle does not penetrate any blood vessel, in that case it is withdrawn and redirected. The injection is completed, the twitch is removed and animal allowed to stand quietly for 10 minutes, and after this the limb is tested for sensation by pricking with a pin or a needle. Any response to pricking around the coronet and heel indicates failure to block the nerve on that side. One indication of sensation is sufficient to prove this. About 2.5 to 5 ml. 2% lignocaine HCl is injected over each nerve. In the hind limb the technique is similar, except that not only must the animal be twitched, but the forelimb should also be necessarily raised, in addition if the operation is to be carried out with the animal standing on the affected limb. The skin and deeper tissues on the anterior aspect of the hind fetlock and pastern are innervated by terminal branches of the deep peroneal (anterior tibial) nerve. The indications for the methods are much less common than in the forelimb.

An alternative site for injection in both the fore and hind limbs is where the nerve courses over the upper part of the fetlock. Although the nerve divides into three branches at about this point the injection of 2 - 3 ml. of lignocaine solution medially and laterally still produces a complete palmar/plantar block. An advantage of this site is that when the limb is held up and the fetlock joint flexed, the nerves and their associated vessels can be palpated and thus their accurate location is easy.

Indications

1. Location of the site of lameness: Palmar/plantar block is invaluable aid to diagnosis of the lameness, particularly of the forelimb, in those cases in which visual and manipulative examinations fail to reveal it, or when doubt exists as to the significance of some obvious lesion. If a horse, previously lame, trots sound after bilateral high palmar/plantar block, it is irrefutable evidence that the cause of lameness lies within the area desensitized. In the great majority of cases it is in the foot. Similarly unilateral block may give useful evidence whether an obvious lesion confined to one side of the foot, such as a tread, a corn or a quarter sand crack, is the cause of lameness. In cases of bilateral fore foot lameness, anaesthesia of the more painful limb serves to demonstrate the existence of lameness in the other.

2. To relieve pain and allow rest: Palmar/plantar block is a valuable therapeutic measure in the treatment of actually painful lesions about the foot, for the relief of pain. The animal experiences much needed rest for an hour or so. The practice may be repeated daily for a few days in severe cases.
3. Operative procedures: Palmar/plantar neurectomy may be performed painlessly either in the cast or standing position. Operative procedures about the foot, coronet and heel, such as exposure of the corn or gathered nail-track, partial operations for quitter and sand crack, are greatly facilitated by the procedure. In fact, most operations about the horse's foot are more conveniently performed with the animal standing.

Accidents and complications: While inserting the needle or during injection, if there is a sudden movement by the animal, especially when the animal is not twitched, it leads to the break of the needle. In some animals perineural injection may lead to the irritation of the connective tissue of the leg, and the reaction generally subsides in 48 hours or so. The horse under the influence of plantar block should not be exercised vigorously for incoordinate movement may result in the fractures of bones especially first and third phalangeal bones.

LOW PALMAR/PLANTAR INJECTION: The posterior terminal branch of the palmar and plantar nerve may be subjected to perineural injection in the pastern region. The site for injection is midway between the fetlock joint and the coronet. The posterior border of the first phalanx is located and behind it the tense dorsal edge of the deep flexor tendon is palpated, as the nerve lies immediately dorsal to the tendon, and 2 - 5 ml of local anaesthetic is injected subcutaneously just proximal to the collateral cartilages. The area desensitized is limited to the posterior part of the foot and heel on that side. This block is usually employed (bilaterally) to reduce the margin of error in the diagnosis of navicular disease.

SUBCARPAL PALMAR/PLANTAR INJECTION: The perineural injection is made for the operation of firing the skin over the flexor tendon, and about 5 ml. of lignocaine HCl solution is injected over each palmar/plantar nerve just below the carpus or tarsus, where the nerve is covered by the carpal sheath and the fluid massaged downwards. The desensitization of the area takes place within 15 minutes.

THE OX

The nerve supply of the digit of the ox is much more complex than in the horse and regional analgesia is more difficult to produce. The skin below the carpus and tarsus is tense and the subcutaneous tissue is very fibrous, so that precise location of nerves is not easy. Many workers consider that simple ring block, in which a transverse plane through the whole extremity is infiltrated, is the most reliable way of producing regional analgesia of the digit. However, block of the individual nerves is more elegant.

Nerve block in the forelimb: The dorsal metacarpal nerve is located by palpation at about the middle of the metacarpus, medial to the extensor tendon. The dorsal branch of the ulnar nerve is blocked about 5 cm. above the fetlock on the lateral aspect of the limb, in the groove between the suspensory ligament and the metacarpal bone. At this point the volar branch of the ulnar nerve may also be blocked, the two nerves being respectively situated in front of, and behind the suspensory ligament.

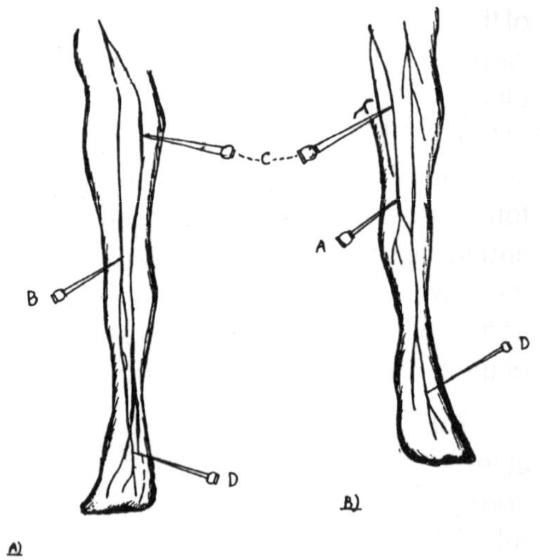

Fig. 31: Needle placement for blocking the Musculocutaneous (A), Ulnar (B), Median (C), and Axial digital III and IV (D) Nerves of the left forelimb in cattle

The axial palmar aspect of digits may be rendered analgesic by a single injection in the midline just above the fetlock. The lateral branch of the median nerve also gets desensitized before it divides. The medial branch of the median nerve is blocked on the inside of the limb in the groove between the suspensory ligament and the flexor tendon about 5 cm. above the fetlock. The median nerve is blocked higher up the limb before the nerve divides. However, at this point the nerve lies beneath the artery and vein (Fig 31).

THE DOG

In the dog the cutaneous branch of radial nerve is divided into a ramus ulnaris on the dorsal aspect of the fore arm below the elbow joint. The ramus ulnaris or the lateral branch passes to the fore arm towards the paw and divides at the end of the metacarpus into branches for the second to fifth digit. A ramus medialis proceeds on the dorsal aspect of the fore arm and innervates the first and second digits. The lateral aspect of the dorsal metacarpus is innervated by lateral cutaneous branch. The cutaneous branch of musculo-cutaneous nerve lies directly in front of the upper arm. The cutaneous nerve runs dorsomedially to the carpus and innervates the skin of the lower arm together with ulnar and median nerves. The ulnar nerve lies on the medial aspect of the humerus. It passes distally to divide at the carpus into deep and superficial rami. The deep branch innervates the first and fourth digits. The superficial ramus innervates the metacarpal pad and the fifth digit. The medial nerve passes from medial side of the humerus to the posterior surface of the fore arm. The median and ulnar nerves innervate together the volar and medial aspects of the fore arm, carpus, metacarpus and digital pads.

Infiltration of radial nerve: The radial nerve can be palpated at the elbow joint by raising a skin fold and the nerve feels like a cord. The needle is inserted at this site, near the nerve and 2 to 3 ml of 2% lignocaine HCl is injected. The area desensitized is dorsal surface of the fore arm, carpus and the digits.

Infiltration of the median, ulnar and musculocutaneous nerves: The site is the point where three nerves are adjacent to each other at a junction of middle and distal third of the humerus. The medial surface of humerus is palpated, since the nerves are passing over it. The needle is inserted towards the humerus at a point 5 to 8 cm above the elbow joint and 3 to 4 ml of 2% local anaesthetic solution is injected. The area desensitized is the distal half of the upper arm, medial aspect of the lower arm, carpus and volar aspects of digits. With this block there is simultaneous anaesthesia of the carpal and digital extensors.

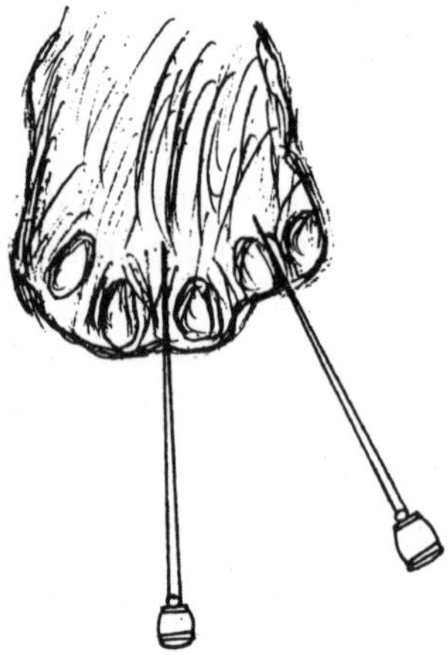

Fig. 32: Injection of the digital nerves in a dog

Infiltration of digital nerves: The digital nerves are approached lateral and medial to the first phalanx of the digit to be rendered analgesic. A fine needle is introduced subcutaneously on each side of the digit (Fig. 32) and 2 ml of local analgesic solution is injected on each aspect.

Intravenous regional analgesia (IVRA): "Venous anaesthesia" was reported by Bier in 1908. However, the technique has widely been used only after 1970 in canine surgery.

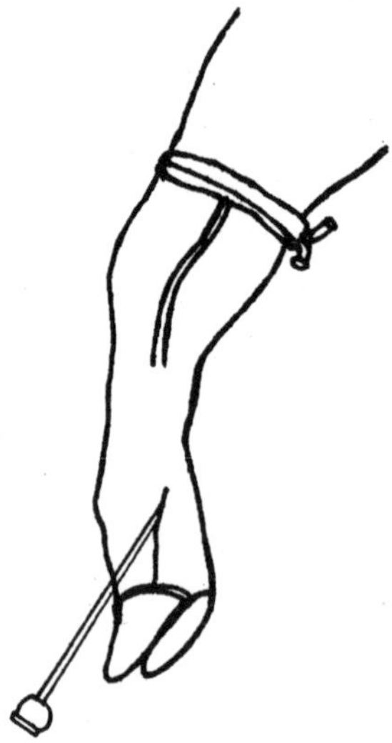

Fig. 33: Needle placement for intravenous regional analgesia

A small needle or catheter is inserted into a vein at the distal extremity of a limb. The limb is exanguinated, usually with an Esmarch bandage, a tourniquet is inflated or tied to occlude the arterial blood supply at the top of the limb and local analgesic solution is injected via the needle or catheter. Analgesia of the limb up to lower limit of the tourniquet courses on rapidly, and when the tourniquet is released it wears off with almost equal rapidity. Up to 30 ml of 2% lingocaine hydrochloride (without adrenaline) is injected in adult cattle. IVRA is certainly safe for periods up to 1 ¼ hours. The mode of action of this technique is unclear but it seems to be both safe and simple for operations of the digits, especially in ruminants (amputation of digits, removal of interdigital hyperplastic lesions and treatment of infection of foot) and in dogs unfit for general anaesthesia because of a full stomach or intercurrent disease. The good analgesia and the bloodless field are appreciated by the surgeon (Fig. 33).

BRACHIAL PLEXUS BLOCK

Cow: The brachial plexus block is induced by a single injection of local anaesthetic in the vicinity of brachial plexus. It is a simple and safe method of attaining regional anaesthesia of the fore limb. The anaesthesia produced is from the elbow joint distally. Motor paralysis however is also produced. The technique has been described by Nutt (1962) in dogs.

The nerves of the fore limbs are derived from the ventral roots of the sixth to eighth cervical and first and second thoracic nerves, and they pass over the lateral surface of the middle third of the first rib beneath the shoulder. The nerves overlap with each other and are well embedded in fat. In the distal quarter of the first rib the large blood vessels are present, which must be avoided.

Technique: In the animals the first rib may be located easily. It should be palpated between the shoulder and the neck, with the limb turned backwards and the head and neck turned to the opposite side. A 20 gauge 16 cm needle is inserted posteriorly in a horizontal and slightly ventral direction until its point contacts the flat surface of the first rib. Here 10 to 15 ml of 2% lignocaine are administered. The needle is slightly withdrawn and readjusted distally along the rib and equal quantity of the anaesthetic deposited. This process is continued until a band of anaesthetic 5 to 8 cm long has been injected along the rib distal to the initial site. A careful check must be made (by aspiration) to ensure no brachial vessel located adjacent to the distal third of the first rib has not been punctured. The area of desensitization includes whole limb from elbow down.

Dog: With the dog standing on all four legs, the triangular area bounded by the anterior border of the supraspinatus muscle, the chest wall and the dorsal border of the brachiocephalicus muscle, is clipped and prepared for injection. The brachial plexus block can also be performed on the recumbent or standing dog. The animal's head is held away from the side to be injected and the depression in the centre of the clipped area is palpated and the first rib blocked. A 18 gauge, 5 to 6 cm long needle is inserted between the sternum and the shoulder joint, straight through the skin, and is then pushed with care slightly medially to the costochondral junction of the rib. After aspiration to confirm that blood vessel has not been punctured 2 to 5 ml of 2% lignocaine Hcl is injected. The onset of anaesthesia is evident within 10 minutes of injection. There is a gradual loss of motor power, followed by complete relaxation and loss of sensation. The area of desensitization includes fore limb distal to the elbow joint. This type of regional anaesthesia of the limb is particularly suitable for the manipulation of fractures and dislocations on account of complete muscular relaxation in dogs. This technique is also of particular value where general anaesthesia is contraindicated owing to the state of the patient when presented for surgery. However, due care is exercised while performing this technique to avoid intravascular injection, damage to brachial plexus and entry of needle into the thorax thereby introduction of infection into the axilla. It is possible that paraesthesia occurs soon after injection, for some animals chew at the leg.

13 Nerve Blocks of Hind Limb

The innervation is from the tibial and peroneal nerves from the sciatic nerve, a branch of the femoral. The tibial nerve runs between the biceps femoris and semi-tendinosus muscles and directly above the tarsus the tibial nerve divides into the medial and lateral metatarsal nerves, analogous to the metacarpal nerves of the forelimb.

The peroneal nerve, which descends with the tibial nerve through the thigh turns outwards over to the head of the fibula where it divides into superficial and deep branches. The deep branch innervates tarsus, the flexors of the hock and digital extensors. It splits into lateral and medial branches that innervate the periosteum and the skin over both aspects of the metatarsus. The superficial peroneal nerve is very strong and passes to the distal end of the hock where it divides into three branches. The tibial nerve divides at the hock into medial and lateral plantar nerves.

Cattle: Usually epidural anaesthesia facilitates the operations of the hind quarters of cattle and this anaesthesia can be easily obtained. However, the regional anaesthesia of the digits of the hind limb can be produced by two injections. The technique involves blocking the tibial and external popliteal (common peroneal) nerves above the hock. The injections can be carried out in standing animals with very minimum restraint. The leg is not paralyzed and can bear the weight in normal manner. Most of the lower limb is rendered insensitive.

The peroneal nerve is blocked immediately behind the posterior edge of the lateral condyle of the tibia (Fig. 34). The lateral condyle is palpated, and a 3 to 5 cm, 18 gauge needle is inserted through the skin and aponeurotic sheath of the biceps femoris until the point just touches the posterior edge of the

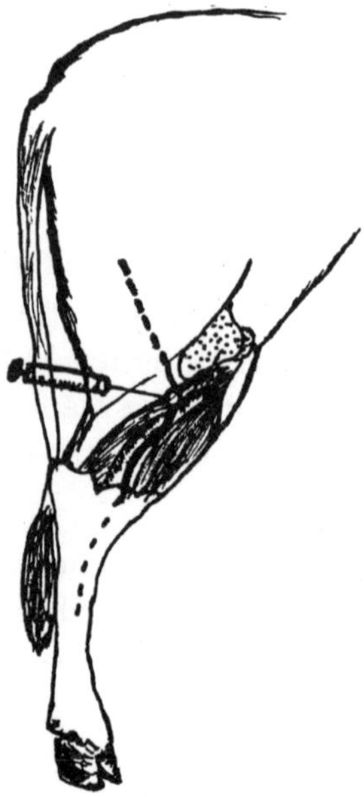

Fig.34: Injection of common peroneal on the outer aspect of limb in Ox

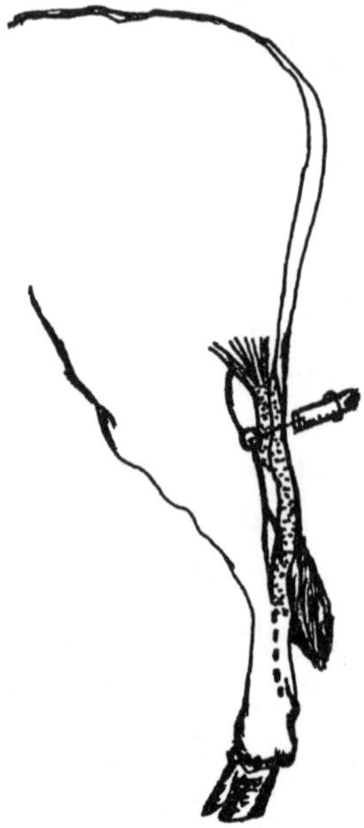

Fig. 35: Injection of the tibial nerve on the inner aspect of limb in Ox

condyle (Collin, 1963). Anaesthesia results 5 to 20 minutes after 20 ml of 2% lidocaine solution is injected.

The tibial nerve is blocked about 10 to 12 cm above the summit of the os calcis on the medial aspect of the limb just in front of the Achilles tendon. The Achilles tendon is grasped between the thumb and index finger of one hand while a needle, about 2.5 cm long, is inserted immediately below the thumb until its point can be felt just under the skin by the index finger. About 15 to 20 ml of local anaesthetic solution are injected at this site and the block takes 5 to 15 minutes to develop. When both nerves are blocked (Fig. 35). There is complete loss of sensation from the fetlock downwards.

The tibial nerve divides into lateral and medial plantar metatarsal nerves and these nerves can be blocked 5 cm above the fetlock in the groove between the suspensory and flexor tendons.

Tibial nerve: In horse injection is made about 15 cm. above the point of the hock, in the groove between the Achilies tendon and deep digital flexors. Palpation of the nerve at this site is facilitated by holding up the foot and slightly flexing the leg although the injection is best made with the limb bearing weight. About 20 ml. of local anaesthetic solution should be injected at this site, deep under the facia.

Peroneal (fibular) nerve: In horse the superficial branch of this nerve is best blocked in the groove between the tendons of the long and lateral extensors 10 cm above the lateral malleolus of the tibia. The needle must be inserted further 2 - 3 cm to penetrate the deep fascia and about 10 ml. of local anaesthetic solution is injected to block the deep branch.

Saphenous nerve: The deposition of 5 ml of local analgesic solution on the dorsal aspect of the median saphenous vein proximal to the tibiotarsal joint will effectively block the saphenous nerve.

Block of the tibial nerve above the hock, and of the deep peroneal (fibular) nerve, desensitizes the posterior metatarsus, the medial and lateral aspects of the fetlock and the whole digit. To produce a complete block distal to the hock, these two nerves must be injected together with the saphenous nerve, the superficial peroneal (fibular) nerve and the posterior cutaneous nerve (a branch of the tibial nerve).

Dog

The common peroneal nerve runs distally underneath the biceps femoris. The nerve divides into superficial and deep rami. The superficial branch runs in the distal half of the tibia along the lateral border of the long digital extensor tendon. It divides again at the tarsus into cutaneous dorsalis medialis nerve to medial surface of tarsus and first digit. At the proximal dorsal border of the metatarsus it divides into three branches for the second to fourth digits. The deep peroneal divides at the tarsus into a lateral branch, that runs to the third and fourth digits, and a medial branch joins the digital branches of superficial peroneal to supply second digit.

The tibialis nerve divides over tarsus into medial and lateral plantar nerves. The medial branch after further division innervates phalanges and digits, while the lateral branches end in the inter-osseous muscles and digits

Saphenous nerve innervates the skin of the medial and dorsal aspects of the thigh as well as the medial aspect of the stifle joint are innervated with one branch. The skin of the medial surface of the tibial region and tarsus is innervated with a second branch. Anaesthesia of the hind quarters is better achieved by epidural anaesthesia, which is easier to perform and more certain of producing complete anaesthesia of the hind quarter

However, anaesthesia of the hind limb from the hock can be produced by infiltration of the tibial and peroneal nerve. Additional anaesthesia of the saphenous nerve renders the skin insensitive over the whole medial aspect of the leg. The saphenous nerve is a branch of the femoral nerve and motor to the sartorius muscle and sensory to the medial surface of the thigh, and leg. It can be reached in the femoral triangle as it runs distally just cranial to the femoral artery. Using the arterial pulse as a landmark, one makes an injection of 2 ml of 2% lidocaine anterior to the artery, being careful to prevent intravascular injection.

The peroneal nerve, a terminal branch of the sciatic nerve, supplies the flexors of the hock and extensors of the digits. It is sensory to the dorsal aspect of the tibial region, hock, and paw. It passes laterally, under cover of the biceps femoris around the fibula just below its head. It can be infiltrated by injecting 2 ml of 2% lidocaine just posterior and dorsal to the head of fibula.

The tibial nerve is the other terminal branch of sciatic. It is motor to the extensors of the hock and flexors of the digits and supplies sensation to the plantar surface of the paw. It can be blocked just above the stifle joint by inserting the needle from behind into the popliteal space between the two heads of the gastrocnemius muscle 2 ml of 2% lidocaine are injected.

EPIDURAL AND CAUDAL BLOCK

It is brought about by the deposition of local analgesic solution between the duramater and periosteum of the spinal canal (epidural space). The anaesthetic solution remains outside the duramater and desensitizes the caudal roots after they emerge from the dura. In most of the animal species the spinal cord ends in the region of the last lumbar vertebra but the meningeal sac is continued as far as third or fourth sacral segment in domestic animals. It is why caudal analgesia in large domestic animals is made safely through the space between arches of the first and second coccygeal vertebrae, i.e., beyond the termination of the spinal cord and its meninges. The spinal cord terminates at the cranial end of the third sacral vertebra as conus medullaris in cow calves and at the junction of the sixth and seventh lumbar vertebrae of the dog.

It is now customary to classify analgesia as epidural (formerly referred to as 'anterior' or 'high') and caudal (formerly 'posterior' or 'low'), according to distance forward the analgesic solution spreads and thus the extent of the area in which sensory and motor paralysis subsequently develops. This will depend chiefly on the volume of solution injected, although the concentration and diffusibility of the drug and the rate of absorption also play a part. If the motor control of the hind limbs is uninfluenced, the block is referred to as a 'caudal block'. 'Epidural block' implies that some degree of interference with the control of the hind limbs is present.

Epidural/caudal block in the bovine species is indicated whenever analgesia of the perineal area, tail or ventral mid-line is desired. Common reasons for administering epidural/ caudal analgesia to the female are (i) to relieve pain in the caudal genital tract while a dystokia is being relieved; (ii) to allow surgery to be performed on the perineal structures (such as repair of third degree lacerations), to facilitate closure of the vulvar lips by Caslick's surgery; and (iii) to relieve straining while uterine or vaginal prolapses are being corrected. In the male, the anaesthesia achieved with epidural block extends forwards to the end of the prepuce and includes the skin of the scrotum. The testicles and penis are not anaesthetized. If larger amount of potent anaesthetic agents is injected into the epidural space, temporary paralysis of the hind leg may occur. This is due to the anaesthetic agent flowing cranially in the epidural space to the level of the motor trunks serving the legs. Some practitioners intentionally use this effect as means of restraining and anaesthetizing for ventral mid-line surgery in both male and female cattle.

Technique: The site of injection should be prepared by clipping or shaving the hair, and site should be thoroughly scrubbed with an antiseptic detergent, and an antiseptic should be applied on the site. The lack of aseptic regimen during the administration of regional or local block leads to local infection or abscessation and delayed healing. The epidural anaesthesia is usually easiest to achieve while the animal is standing and restrained in a squeezed chute. Sacrococcygeal space or first intercoccygeal space is the site where injection is made for epidural anaesthesia. The site of injection is identified by alternately elevating and lowering the tail with one hand, and with other hand determining where the vertebral joints are located by palpating the depression and movement between the vertebrae. The location at which the tail movement ceases in young to middle aged animals is the sacrococcygeal articulation. In older animals, the sacrococcygeal articulation is ossified and the first intercoccygeal articulation is the joint at which tail movement ceases. Using a small gauge needle, a small amount of anaesthetic is injected into the skin over the site. This renders the animal less sensitive to subsequent passage of the large needle.

The 16 to 18 gauge needle is passed downwards between the vertebrae at a 10 degree angle caudally from perpendicular. The needle is inserted directly on the mid-line and usually to a depth of about 1.5 to 2 inches, depending on the size, fattiness, and thickness of the tail. Occasionally, the needle strikes the artery or vein ventral to the epidural space, and blood flows from the needle. This is of little concern. It indicates that the needle is near the proper site for injection, or just below the epidural space. The needle should be slightly retracted before its insertion continues. The syringe is attached to the needle and the anaesthetic solution is injected. If the epidural space has been entered, introduction of the fluid is easy and resistance is almost nil. With the needle in any other position, deposition of fluid is quite difficult. The required amount of anaesthetic solution varies among products and with the depth of anaesthesia needed for the procedure to be performed. Usually lignocaine Hcl (2%) at the rate of 0.02 mg/kg body weight (5 to 6 ml) or 0.04 mg /kg body weight (10 to 12 ml) procaine (2%) is used to anaesthetise the tail and perineal area of the cattle. This dose should allow the animal to remain standing. If recumbency is desired, 10 to 20 ml of lignocaine (2%) or 20 to 50 ml of procaine (2%) may be given.

The progress of anaesthesia begins with the loss of sensation at the tip of the tail almost immediately, advances to root, then spreads to the perineum. Anaesthesia is maximum in about15 minutes. At that time the area of desensitized skin extends upwards to the middle of the sacral spine and downwards over the perineum and inner aspects of the thighs. The duration of epidural anaesthesia varies with the anaesthetic agent used. Usually, anaesthesia lasts for about 60 minutes when procaine is used and 90 minutes in respect of lignocaine. If the solution contains epinephrine, the duration of anaesthesia will be approximately doubled (Fig.36).

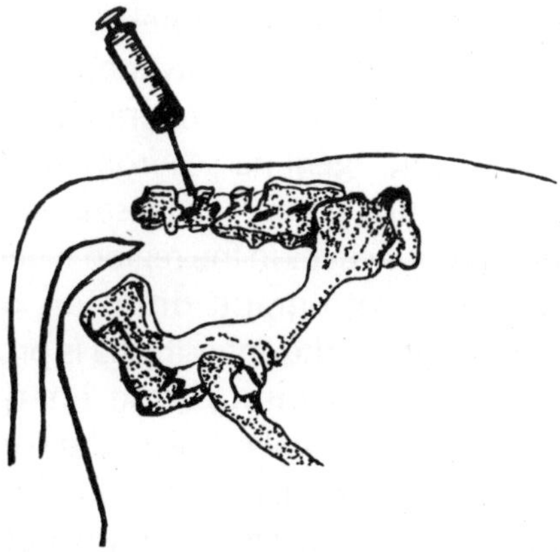

Fig. 36: Caudal epidural injection in cattle. Insertion of the needle into first intercoccygeal space

Lumbar epidural analgesia: Injection into the epidural space in the lumbar region has been employed to produce analgesia of a number of the segments in cattle. By careful control of the dose of local analgesic injected it is possible to produce a belt of analgesia around the animal's trunk without interfering with the control of the hind-limbs. Arthur's technique involves insertion of the needle just to the right of the lumbar spinous processes on a line 1.5 cm behind the cranial edge of the second lumbar transverse process. Although it is not an easy technique to perform, it is valuable for operations about the flank and udder.

Mechanism of action in epidural anaesthesia: Conduction anaesthesia by the injection of local anaesthetic drugs into epidural space of the spinal canal is a well-established technique in veterinary and human medicine. However, the principle site of neural uptake of drug remains a matter of conjecture. The sites suggested for action of local anaesthetic drugs after epidural injection are the spinal nerve roots within the spinal canal, the mixed nerves in the paravertebral spaces and the neuritis and the spinal cord. The two preferential paths through which the local anaesthetic agent passes from the epidural to the subarachnoid space during epidural anaesthesia in cows are dural passage via dural root sleeves in the region where the dorsal and ventral roots fuse and retrograde diffusion of local anaesthetic across perineurium. The anaesthesia is produced after local anaesthetic agent diffuses through the intervertebral foramina, thereby blocking the spinal nerves at the paravertebral sites. It is probably a non-essential feature confined to young subjects with freely patent foramina. It is unlikely to occur to any significant extent in older subjects and with small volumes of solution.

The caudal epidural anaesthesia in large animals is due to nerve block as the spinal cord and its meninges extend posteriorly in the spinal canal and terminate at the cranial end of the third sacral vertebra as conus medullaris.

Anatomy: The epidural space lies within the vertebral canal and surrounds the spinal cord and its enveloping membranes (spinal piamater, arachnoid and duramater). It is bounded internally by the duramater (a continuation of meningeal layer of the duramater of brain). Externally, it is limited by vertebral bodies and arches, intervertebral discs and associated ligaments. In the cranium the endosteal and meningeal layers of duramater are closely united, but below the foramen magnum the two layers separate, the outer becoming the periosteal lining of spinal canal and inner forming the spinal duramater. The periosteum of the vertebrae is a continuation of the outer layer of the cerebral dura and joins with the internal meningeal layer of the duramater at the foramen magnum. The epidural space terminates at this point. The epidural space between the dural tube and the walls of the spinal canal is a potential space filled with fat, blood vessels and lymphatics. The space also contains spinal nerve roots, spinal membranes within which are the cord and associated spinal fluid and areolar tissue in which the cord is suspended. The dural tube, with its lateral prolongation covering each pair of spinal nerve roots, extends from the foramen magnum to the middle of the sacral region. Major blood vessels of significance with the canal are the paired vertebral venous sinuses, which extend longitudinally along the floor of vertebral canal. Since they anastomose freely with other veins draining the trunk and with the azygos vein, they provide an alternative route for venous return which bypasses canal. Besides these vessels, branches of cervical, intercostal, lumbar, and ilio-lumbar arteries enter the cava through intervertebral foramen. Epidural anaesthesia can be classified into cranial or caudal according to the distance that the anaesthetic solution spreads, and extent of the area in which sensory and motor paralysis develops. Caudal epidural anaesthesia implies that motor control of hind legs is not effected.

Horses: Lumbar, lumbosacral, or even caudal epidural anaesthesia is rarely used because of the temperament of the horses, the possibility of the injuring during recovery, and the difficulties of prolonged restraint. The amount of anaesthesia injected is small, so that only posterior blockade is induced, and the animal remains standing, with appropriate restraint such as stocks, chemical sedation such as xylazine may also be needed. The site, technique and indications are same as in bovines.

In sheep and goats indications and site are similar to those for bovines caudal epidural anaesthesia, injection being made through the sacrococcygeal space, at the rate of 0.02 mg/kg body weight of 2% lignocaine.

In dog the epidural anaesthesia is indicated in the following situations, caesarean section, ovariohysterectomy, castration, reduction of rectal prolapse, caudectomy, mammectomy, excision of skin tumours of the hind quarters, fracture repair of the hind quarter, relaxation of the abdomen to facilitate palpation, repair of nerves of the hind quarters.

Preanaesthetic administration of a sedative/tranquilliser aids in restraint during injection. The area over lumbosacral space is clipped and scrubbed with surgical soap and antiseptic solution is applied. The dog is held in a sternal position by an assistant. Immediately posterior to the spinous process of L_7, the lumbosacral space is identified and a 20 gauge needle is introduced. After subcutaneous weal of anaesthetic, the site is raised. The needle is inserted through the intervertebral ligament and introduced until it touches the floor of the vertebral canal. It is now withdrawn slightly and anaesthetic solution injected without any resistance over a period of 15 to 30 second period, otherwise vomiting and convulsions may result. The analgesia is achieved within 5 - 10 minutes if lignocaine (2% with 1:2,00,000 adrenaline) is used but within 15 - 30 minutes if bupivacaine (0.75%) is used. Lignocaine block usually lasts for 1.5 - 2 hours and bupavicaine block lasts for 5 - 6 hours. The latter is preferred if postoperative analgesia is required. The local analgesic solution should be warmed by placing ampules in hot water before use.

The advantages of epidural analgesia over general anaesthesia in dogs include the absence of respiratory worries when dealing with the brachycephalic dogs, the completeness of muscle relaxation, the absence of straining when traction is applied to peritoneum and the absence of depression of the fetuses in caesarian section. The tail relaxes, followed by anal sphincter, and soon the rare quarters collapse.

Caudal continuous epidural analgesia: Corning (1885) was the first to report the use of epidural anaesthesia in a dog. Lemmon (1940) was credited as the first to describe a method for continuous spinal anaesthesia in man, in which a malleable needle was introduced into the subarachnoid space. Continuous epidural anaesthesia has been well described in the dog (Kide, 1971). Its use has also been reported as segmental lumbar epidural analgesia in the cow (Skarda and Muir, 1979) and continuous subarachnoid analgesia has been described in horse by Skarda and Muir (1982). A technique for continuous caudal epidural anaesthesia was developed by Hussain and Kumar (1989). Operations around the perineal area and tail of cattle are usually performed in the standing animal, using caudal epidural anaesthesia. Due to the development of more sophisticated surgical techniques the operative time often extends beyond the duration of anaesthesia. Repetition of epidural anaesthesia in most cases requires disruption of the surgical field. Continuous caudal epidural anaesthesia allows easy access to a catheter preplaced into epidural space for re-administration of an anaesthetic agent without disturbance of the surgical area, break in asepsis, or inconvenience to the surgeon.

A technique for continuous caudal epidural anaesthesia in the buffalo calves was developed in the experimental study. A technique of continuous caudal epidural anaesthesia was performed in each animal to induce anaesthesia of the perineal area. Repeated doses of anaesthetic were administered immediately upon the detection of return of sensation to the perineal area. Sensation was determined by application of haemostats to the anus, vulva and perineal area. The site of injection prepared was first intercoccygeal space. A 16 gauge spinal needle about 3 inches long, that was manually curved at is distal end was used.

Each animal was restrained in a trevis. The tail is gripped about six inches from its base and elevated "pump handle fashion." The first obvious articulation posterior to sacrum indicates the sacrococcygeal space. The sacrococcygeal is the preferable site for the introduction of the tubing through the tough needle. The space between the first and second coccygeal vertebrae may be used, but it has been found that the former site better facilitates the placement of the tubing. The site is prepared for injection, using standard aseptic procedures. To minimise response to insertion of epidural needle, anaesthesia at the injection site is induced by subcutaneous infiltration of 1 ml of 2% lignocaine HCl. A hypodermic needle is used to make a skin puncture that facilitates the passage of the 16 gauge spinal needle that is manually curved and blunted at its distal end. The spinal needle with stillete in place is inserted through the puncture wound in the skin, making sure the orifice of the needle is directed downward at an angle of 10°. Handy pressure is applied to the hub of the needle, thrusting it vertically until it touched the ventral floor of the canal and then it is withdrawn slightly dorsally. The stillete is removed from the needle. A small amount of local anaesthetic solution is injected to ascertain the location of the needle. Once the epidural space is entered, introduction of fluid becomes easy and virtually no resistance is encountered. An indwelling catheter of No 47 (0.036 cm O.D.) is threaded through the lumen of the needle and advanced cranially approximately for a distance of 2 to 4 inches, beyond the tip of the needle, into the vertebral canal. Ease of catheter introduction and failure of aspiration of blood indicates location within the vertebral canal. The needle is slowly withdrawn over the tubing, while the tubing is held firmly about half an inch beyond the hub. The needle is withdrawn in short repeated semi-rotating motions. After the needle is completely withdrawn, a 23 gauge half inch needle is inserted into the epidural space. To keep the apparatus firmly anchored, two pieces of adhesive tape are applied. The first anchoring tape is applied over the catheter about half inch anterior to the site of insertion and adhered to the adjacent haired areas. A second tape is applied to the end of the tubing to the dorsal concave portion of the pelvis, approximately two inches lateral to the spines of the sacrum and approximately three inches posterior to the point of the tuber saccrale of the illium. After every administration, the outer end of the catheter is sealed by application of flame at the tip to prevent entrance of infection into the epidural space. The sealed end is cut-off for the next injection and again sealed.

The technique of continuous epidural anaesthesia has been used as an aid in treatment of prolapse of the rectum, prolapse of vagina, necrotic vulvo-vaginitis and obstetrical cases. Through the use of continuous epidural anaesthesia cases of threatened prolapse of the rectum and vagina have been prevented.

A single epidural injection of procaine HCl 2%, or lignocaine hydrochloride 2%, or bupivacaine hydrochloride 2% produced a zone of anaesthesia, which lasts from one to four hours depending upon the agents chosen. The duration of anaesthesia is prolonged by intermittent injection of local anaesthetic agents through an indwelling catheter. Bupivacaine hydrochloride 0.5% which is having prolonged duration of action among all available local anaesthetic agents, is used for continuous epidural anaesthesia, however, the maximum duration of epidural anaesthesia does not exceed 14 hours with four repeated injections. The repeated injections of local anaesthetic agents result into a tolerance to these anaesthetic agents and duration of anaesthesia is not proportional to the amount injected. Such an exponential reduction of response with each successive injection of local anaesthetic agents like procaine and lignocaine hydrochloride was also observed in buffalo calves by Hussain and Kumar (1993). The existence of tachyphylaxis phenomenon makes the use of continuous epidural infusion of local anaesthetic agents a difficult proposition and invalidates the use of continuous epidural blockade for anaesthesia of longer period of time.

There are situations where the tenesmus due to chronic preolapse of vagina/uterus in animals persists for days together, and straining recommences after the effects of the caudal block have worn off. The epidural anaesthesia in such cases is required for days.

Alcohol block: Amyl alcohol (98%) at a dose of 0.01 mg/kg preceded by 2% lignocaine hydrochloride at the dose rate of 0.025 mg/kg epidurally has been used to control straining/tenesmus in cows and buffaloes with vaginal prolapse (Hussain and Kumar, 1989). In these animals local anaesthetic solution had failed to prevent recurrence of tenesmus and prolapse. The tenesmus was stopped in about 1 minute following the alcohol injection and did not recur. The animals lactated and ate normally through the period following prolonged alcohol block. However, the animals could not elevate their tail or react to painful stimuli to the tail and perineal region, even 21 days after the injection. About this time, sensation was beginning to return to the perineal region. Urination and defecation could be performed without serious difficulty.

The epidural administration of amyl alcohol procedure should be used as a last resort. This block is generally irreversible and associated with adverse effects. But in cases where there is persistent tenesmus and therapeutic options or alternatives fail to prevent recurrence of tenesmus, amyl alcohol block is of great value in combating the recurrence of tenesmus in such cases.

Epidural narcosis: The discovery of specific opiate receptors within the central nervous system in the early 1970s led to better appreciation of the selective action of the opiates. It is now known that there are several types of opiate receptors, and their anatomic locations within the central nervous system have been described. The analgesic actions of opiates appear to be due, at least in part, to the close association of the receptors with major regions in the spinal cord and brain involved in pain sensation. The two most studied locations in recent years have been (i) a local system within the dorsal horn of the spinal cord, modulating on the substantia gelatinosa, and (ii) descending system from the brain stem to the dorsal horn, such as the periaqueductal grey.

Morphine: Morphine, like local analgesics, when injected into the epidural space reaches their site of action by diffusion across the dura. The morphine, once in the CSF and bathing the spinal cord, spreads into the cord to the opiate receptors. Morphine, a polar hydrophilic agent, penetrates the dura slowly and clearance from CSF.

Epidural administration of morphine sulphate at the rate of 3 mg/kg body weight with premedication of atropine sulphate at the rate of 0.02 mg/kg and chlorpromazine hydrochloride at the rate of 2 mg/kg body weight in dogs produce effective surgical anaesthesia lasting for 90 to 150 minutes. The anaesthesia facilitates various surgical operations in dogs. Epidural morphine also provides post-operative analgesia lasting for 10 to 12 hours in dogs. When they are used by epidural injection, care must be taken to ensure that the solution used does not contain a preservative, for this may damage nerves.

Xylazine: Xylazine is used for its α_2-agonistic effects to achieve caudal epidural anaesthesia in cattle and horses. Although xylazine will provide epidural anaesthesia of 2 to 3 hours and does not cause ataxia at clinical doses. The epidural administration of a combination of lignocaine and xylazine to horses results in rapid onset and prolonged duration of anaesthesia. The dose of xylazine given epidurally should not exceed 0.24 mg/kg, otherwise it may cause ataxia.

14 Use of Preanaesthetics in Animals

Preanaesthetic drugs are given to the animals for multiple reasons. The premedication with sedatives moderately depresses the central nervous system. The sedatives are given for producing calming effect of conscious animals for routine examination, diagnostic procedures, and for premedication before general anaesthesia. The preanaesthetic antisialgouge agents are used to reduce the secretion of the salivary glands and mucous glands of the respiratory tract and maintain a free air way. These agents also reduce gastric and intestinal motility and prevent vomiting while the animal is under anaesthesia. They block the vago-vagal reflex, thus preventing cardiac slowing or arrest and reduce pain, struggling of the animal during the recovery period. Many preanaesthetic agents are capable of producing analgesia, sedation or narcosis in conjunction with local anaesthetic in animals to a degree that will facilitate many surgical procedures to be carried out without general anaesthesia. Their use in combination with local anaesthetic helps to restrain and ally apprehension during surgical procedures. Employing such combination sometimes helps avoid the dangers of general anaesthesia.

There are many types of drugs used as preanaesthetic agents. The commonly employed drugs for premedication include atropine, hyoscine, sedatives, narcotics, tranquilizers, opiate and non-opiate analgesics and their combinations.

Atropine sulfate: This is an alkaloid that is obtained from *Atropa belladonna* (deadly night shade). It is potent antisialogogue and vagolytic and is effective in countering the unwanted muscaranic response to anticholinesterase. It is given by injection 15 - 20 minutes before administration of anaesthetic agents.

Dosage: In dogs 0.02 to 0.05 mg/kg, in cat doses of up to 0.3 mg (approximately 0.1 mg/kg for an adult cat) are perfectly safe and in horse 20 to 60 mg/kg. Pigs may be given from 0.3 to

1.8 mg according to size. The atropine sulphate is supplied in a solution containing 0.6 mg/ml. A large animal preparation containing 10 mg/ml is now available. Atropine should not be administered in ruminants. It does not stop the flow of saliva but make the secretion more viscid and thus more difficult to remove from respiratory tract.

Hyoscine (scopolamine): It is an alkaloid resembling atropine obtained from the shrub henbane (*Hyoscyamus niger*). The peripheral actions of hyoscine resemble those of atropine. It blocks action of acetylcholine liberated at parasympathetic post ganglionic nerve endings and in fact at any site where this exhibits muscarine-like effects. It is more potent antisialogogue but less effective as a vagolytic so that its effect on heart rate is less than atropine. In horses, hyoscine may produce considerable excitement. It has been used as the hydrobromide for premedication in dogs in doses of 0.2 to 0.4 mg and it is often used in combination with papaveretum (omnopon-scopolamine, Roche). This standard preparation contains 20 mg of papaveretum with 0.4 mg of hyoscine per milliliter of solution.

Glycopyrrolate: It has recently been introduced as a quaternary ammonium anticholinergic agent with powerful and prolonged antisialogogue activity. It is 5 times as potent antisialgouge as atropine. Glycopyrrolate does not readily cross the blood-brain barrier which means it has little central action. Therefore, it causes less effect on vision than atropine or hyoscine. Thus it is anticholinergic of choice in horses and cats. It has been used in veterinary practice in doses of 0.01 to 0.02 mg/kg.

Commonly used tranquilizers/sedatives/hypnotics/ analgesics: They include phenothiazines, butyrophenones, benzodiazepines, narcotics, non-narcotics, dissociative agents and their combinations.

Phenothiazine derivatives: The predominant class of tranquilizers used in animals is the phenothiazines. They may cause depression of the brain stem that depresses alertness, yielding sedation. Relieve anxiety and restrain refractory animals during examination of large animals during transportation. Prevent animals from licking wounds or chewing bandages and splints. Phenothiazines have been valuable in the chemical restraint of animals for various diagnostic and clinical procedures. Their value in quieting and calming unfriendly and apprehensive animals has been beneficial in the preparation of animals for neuroleptanalgesia and general anaesthesia. Phenothiazine derivatives potentiate the effect of analgesics, hypnosis and local and general anaesthetic. In all ruminants, the phenothiazines relax the gastro-oesophageal junction, and increase the risk of regurgitation of·ruminal contents. They are contraindicated in epidural anaesthetic procedures because they potentiate the arterial hypotensive effects of local analgesia. The arterial hypotension is due to central nervous system depression and peripheral-adrenergic receptor blockade, but it is usually mild if moderate doses are used. However, in the presence of hypovolaemia from any cause, hypotension may be severe and circulatory failure may occur when the drug is used alone or followed by local and general anaesthesia. Intravenous fluids with balanced electrolytes add volume to the dilated vascular bed and increase venous return to allow maintenance of cardiac output. They are contraindicated in cardiovascular diseases and in breeding stallions. The phenothiazine derivatives are detoxified in liver and excreted through the urine. Commonly used phenothiazine tranquilizers are the following.

Chlorpromazine hydrochloride (largactil): Chlorpromazine hydrochloride is a powerful sedative and potent gangliolytic and adrenolytic drug. It has a wide margin of safety. It produces marked antiemetic, antipyretic, hypothermic and peripheral antiadrenaline effect. It is very useful in cattle and is considered a satisfactory agent for sedation in cattle. However, it should not be given intravenously in cattle as it has shown the signs of idiosyncrasy. Chlorpromazine should not be used as a sole sedative in equines because it can cause excitement, muscle weakness, ataxia and knuckling of the hind quarters. It was extensively used in dogs. It prevents narcotic excitement during recovery from barbiturates.

In veterinary practice it has largely been replaced by acepromazine and propionyl promazine. Its actions and side-effects are similar to those of acepromazine, but it is less potent, has a longer duration of action and produces relatively less sedation. The dose for all species lies between 0.5 and 2.0 mg/kg body weight when administered intramuscularly. Orally 5 mg/kg body weight may be given in dogs only. In small animals collapse of the third eyelid and wrinkling of the face provides an indication of the point when further procedure may commence. In large animals 5% solution and in small animals 0.5% concentration are used intramuscularly. In small animals 2.5% solution is used intravenously. In all species it is usual to allow about 5 minutes to elapse after intravenous injection and 40 minutes or more after intramuscular injection. Oral dosing may not give maximum effects for up to three hours after dosing.

Triflupromazine hydrochloride (siquil): It is a potent nervous system depressant and can cause marked sedation and suppression of sympathetic nervous system. It is 2 to 3 times more potent than chlorpromazine. It intensifies and prolongs the action of barbiturates and other narcotic and anaesthetics. Its rapid intravenous injection causes hypotension and sometimes cardiovascular collapse. In dogs 1 to 2 mg/kg body weight is given intravenously and 2 to 4 mg/kg intramuscularly. In cattle, triflupromazine is given at the rate of 0.1 mg/ kg body weight intravenously and 0.2 mg/kg body weight intramuscularly. In horses it is given at the rate of 0.2 to 0.3 mg/kg body weight, however the maximum dose should not exceed 100 mg. In sheep and goats, 0.1 to 0.2 mg/kg body weight is given intramuscularly or intravenously up to a maximum of 40 mg. The drug is supplied as an aqueous solution in 5 ml multiple dose vials providing 20 mg/ml. Vials should be protected from exposure to light. If a solution has become any darker than light amber or is discoloured in any other way it should not be used.

Promazine hydrochloride (sparine): It is frequently used in large animal anaesthesia and is less hypotensive and has fewer side-effects than chlorpromazine. It is used as an ataractic in all the domestic animals. It can be given intravenously to horses and cattle without provoking panic. The duration of action is comparatively shorter, and is about 2 hours. In horses, cattle, sheep, goats and dogs most satisfactory doses are about 0.5 mg/kg intravenously or 1.0 mg/kg intramuscularly.

Acetylpromazine maleate (Acepromazine): It is the tranquilizer of choice in equines and in other animals. It is the most potent of phenothiazine derivatives, and produces a central nervous depression with sedation, muscular relaxation and reduction in spontaneous activity. It is effective in preventing cardiac arrythmias as it provides a protective effect against epinephrine induced ventricular arrhythmias. The onset of action occurs within 15 to 20 minutes following intravenous administration and it lasts for approximately 2 hours. The maximum effects are seen within 30 to 45 minutes after intramuscular and subcutaneous injection. Acepromazine is also being used in combination with etorphin as "Large Animals Immobilon". Parenteral doses of acepromazine for sedative and premedicant purposes in most domestic animals are in the range 0.025 - 0.1 mg/kg. In equines 0.044 to 0.088 mg/kg produces quick onset, where 01 mg to 0.3 mg/kg intramuscularly produces sedation for 2 to 3 hours. In dogs and cats 0.03 to 0.05 mg/kg body weight intramuscularly produces good sedation. Dogs of boxer breed are renowned for their liability to "faint" following even small doses of phenothiazine derivatives (e.g., 0.02 mg/kg acepromazine by intramuscular injection).

Propionylpromazine (combelen): The hypnotic effect is greater than chlorpromazine. It is widely used in Scandinavia and Europe. Its antihistaminic property corresponds to that of promazine. It has been used in combination with methadone for general sedation of all species of animals. The dose in equines varies from 0.15 to 0.25 mg/kg, intravenously or intramuscularly. In cattle the recommended dose is 5 to 15 mg/kg body weight intramuscularly. The dose rate in dogs is 0.2 to 0.3 mg/kg body weight that produces sleepiness after 10 minutes, whereas in sheep and goats 0.5 to 1.0 mg/kg intravenously or intramuscularly dose rate is given.

Butyrophenone tranquilizers: The butyrophenone derivatives have been recently introduced in veterinary practice, for their potency and relatively long duration of action. They are mainly used in combination with analgesics as neurolept analgesics in animals. The following are the commonly used derivatives.

Azaperone (stresnil): It is one of the butyrophenone derivatives. It has been used in capture and control of wild species of animals. It can also be used as preanaesthetic agent for controlling the animal for administration of local anaesthetic drugs. In horses 0.4 to 0.8 mg/kg body weight is given intramuscularly for this purpose.

Droperidol (droleptan, dehydrobenzperidol): It is an extremely potent antiemetic and is said to antagonize the respiratory depressant effects of morphine-like compounds. It is mainly used in combination with narcotic fentanyl (Innovar-vet). Clinically, in a low dose droperidol alone appears to have maximum adverse effects on pulmonary function.

The other derivatives include haloanisone, (fluanisone) which imparts similar action when combined with analgesics, as neurolpt analgesic agent.

Benzodiazipine derivatives: They are a group of drugs that exhibit dose-related tranquilizing, sedative and hypnotic properties. The benzodiazepine derivatives have anticonvulsant activity and ability to produce muscle relaxation. The tranquilization is affected in the limbic system of brain, particularly hipocampus whilst muscle relaxation is completely independent of sedation and is due to an action at spinal cord level. Mostly used benzodiazepine derivatives in veterinary practice include diazepam (valium), chlordiazepoxide (librium) and lorazepam (ativan). Diazepam and more recently lorazepam have been used as intravenous or adjunct agents.

Diazepam: The mino tranquilizer diazepam is a benzodiazepinne derivative that has a negligible effect on respiration and circulation. It has calming, muscle relaxation and anticonvulsant effects. It produces CNS depression in brain stem reticular formation. Diazepam is incompatible with aqueous solution leading to precipitation of the active substance. In equines the dose is 1 mg/kg body weight intramuscularly, whereas 0.5 mg/kg body weight intravenously. In cattle, sheep and goat the dose is 0.5 mg/kg body weight intramuscularly, whereas in the dog the dose is 2 mg/kg body weight intramuscularly but intravenously 1 to 1.5 mg/kg body weight. There is an absence of cardiovascular or other side-effects even with larger doses. The onset of action is evident within 5 minutes after intravenous administration whereas 45 minutes are required to produce effect after intramuscular injection. It is commonly used as a component of balanced anaesthesia with narcotics or ketamine at a dose of 0.2 to 0.5 mg/kg intravenously or intramuscularly. Its clinical effect is short-lasting from 15 to 30 minutes under most circumstances. This drug has been used widely in veterinary anaesthesia in recent years. It is particularly useful in anaesthetic combination with other drugs.

Lorazepam (ativan): This is very long-acting benzodiazepine and is 4 times more potent than diazepam. The onset of action is slow and it takes 30 to 40 minutes after intravenous injection and 40 to 50 minutes after oral administration. It is used especially for premedication in cats before administration of saffan and the anaesthesia was prolonged for several hours.

Chlordiazepoxide (librium): It is less potent than diazepam. It has been used in wild animals with good results. The dose varies from 2.2 to 5.0 mg/kg intramuscularly in all wild animals.

Rauwolfia derivatives: The derivatives of this group that are important in veterinary practice include reserpine and metoserpate hydrochloride. Reserpine is an alkaloid obtained from *Rauwolfia serpes*. It has delayed onset of action, however very smaller doses are required to produce calming effect in animals. The dose in dogs varies from 45 μg/kg to 0.25 mg/day and in rabbits 1 to 2 μg daily produces tranquilization and in cattle an intravenous dose of 7 to 7.5 mg/300 kg will produce a satisfactory tranquilization.

Metoserpate hydrochloride: It is used as a tranquilizer for flock treatment of birds. It is used as a one-time treatment for replacement chickens in the flock up to 16 weeks of age, at a dose level of 568.5 mg per gallon of drinking water.

Opoid analgesics: The narcotic analgesics are the most powerful systemic analgesics known. In veterinary practice the narcotic analgesics are used in a number of ways. They are used for the relief of preoperative pain and for the post-operative pain. They are combined with tranquilizers/sedatives for neurolept analgesic and neurolept anaesthetic preparations. They impart their action by combining with opiate receptors in brain and spinal cord. They are metabolized by the liver and excreted in the urine. The non-narcotic analgesic important in veterinary practice are xylazine hydrochloride and pentazocine.

Pentazocine (talwin): It is a non-addicting drug having general effects and its analgesic potency is 16 to 25% to that of morphine. It weakly antagonizes morphine and meperidine. It is agonist/antagonist analgesic that produces minimal sedation and little or no respiratory or cardiovascular depression. It is used in combination with tranquilizers for conducting surgical maneuvers in standing animals. It can be given subcutaneously or intramuscularly before anaesthesia with sedation provided by diazepam 0.2 mg/kg or acetyl promazine 0.05 mg/kg in dogs. It is also beneficial for relief of colic pain in horses. In equines the dose varies from 0.44 to 0.88 mg/kg intravenously or intramuscularly. Two hundred ten to 300 mg of pentazocine combined with 30 mg of acepromazine can be given intravenously to a 500 kg horse.

The narcotic analgesics include the powerful systemic analgesic. These analgesics both stimulate and depress the central nervous system. The depression of central nervous system causes analgesia, sedation, hypnosis, depression of the cough reflex and the action due to stimulation of central nervous system include general excitements are even convulsions. The narcotic analgesics commonly used in veterinary practice include the following agents.

Morphine: It is probably the most powerful naturally occurring analgesic drug. It is used as one of the soluble salts — the sulfate or hydrochloride. It has been used in combination with rompun which masks the undesirable excitatory side-effect of morphine. Morphine is the narcotic analgesic against which all others are compared. The dose of 0.1 to 0.3 mg/kg by intramuscular injection will usually provide good analgesia for about four hours in most species of animals if they are in pain when the drug is given, but in cats it may be safer to restrict the dose to 0.1 mg/kg. Excitement reactions, bradycardia and histamine release are more common when the drug is given by the intravenous route and even after intravenous injection analgesia may not become apparant for some 15 minutes.

Meperidine hydrochloride: It is a synthetic, anticholinergic narcotic. Its analgesic activity is between codeine and morphine. It causes sedation, peristalsis, and histamine release. The onset of action is within 15 to 25 minutes after injection. The dose in equines varies from 1.1 to 4.4 mg/kg intramuscularly or intravenously. Two hundred fifty milligram meperidine hydrochloride may be combined with 25 mg acepromazine and 12.5 ml of this solution can be given intravenously to 500 kg horse to induce analgesia. The dosage in dogs is 1 mg/kg intramuscularly or subcutaneously.

Methadone: It is equipotent to morphine in terms of analgesia. It causes respiratory depression and bradycardia. It may cause salivation and decrease peristalsis. It is widely used as analgesic and sedative in horse. It should be used in combination with phenothiazine tranquillizer in horse to prevent undesirable effects. The dose in equine is 0.11 to 0.22 mg/kg body weight intramuscularly. The dose for the drug is generaly accepted to be 0.25 mg/kg.

Fentanyl: It is a neurolept analgesic. It is 50 times as potent as morphine. It is very short acting. Effective following intravenous, intramuscular and subcutaneous injection, it is also rapidly absorbed across mucous membranes. It has been used to produce complete anaesthesia in dogs. It is used in surgical procedures in animals with local analgesia. It is also used in combination with atropine premedication. It is administered at the dose rate of 1.0mg/9 to 14 kg body weight. Each ml of droperidol-fentanyl (Innovar-vet) contains a mixture of 20 mg/ml droperidol and 0.4 mg/ml fentanyl with 1.0 mg/ml methyl paraben and 0.2 mg/ml propyl paraben as preservatives. Dogs should always receive an anticholinergic to counteract the vagal effect produced by the narcotic unless there is tachycardia before anaesthesia.

Etorphine: It is a very potent derivative of morphine. Its use causes an initial period of excitement. To overcome this excitement, it is combined with phenothiazine tranquilizers and used as neuroleptic analgesic mixture. It is effective at the dose rate of 0.5 mg/500 kg body weight. In anaesthetic practice this very same potency makes it a difficult drug to handle and constitutes a hazard to the anaesthetist. It causes respiratory depression. Effective doses for a very large animal can be desolved in a very small volume of solvent, enabling it to be used in dart gun projectiles for immobilizing wild game animals. It is extremely long acting compound. Its action is usually terminated by the use of diprenorphine.

Buprenorphine (temgesic): It is almost 30 times as potent as morphine and is effective for at least 8 hours, sometimes even longer. Therefore it has a distinct advantage for post-operative analgesia. A combination of buprenorphine with acepromazine prodcuces sedation equal to that of omnopon/acepromazine. Acepromazine (0.05 mg/kg) is mixed in a syringe with b uprenorphine (0.006 mg/kg) and the mixture injected intravenously is more accepted. Buprenorphine is administered at the dose rate of 0.006 mg/kg body weight.

Papavertum (omnopon): It is often used in dogs instead of morphine because it causes less nausea and vomiting than morphine itself. The commercial preparation known as omnopon - scopolamine (Roche) contains 20 mg of omnopon with 0.4 mg of hyoscine and is available as 1 ml ampules. One ampule of this preparation given by intramuscular injection in combination with 3 - 5 mg of acepromazine has been found to make even the largest and most vicious of dogs easy to handle with safety.

Antagonists or reversal agents: Antagonists displace the narcotic from the receptor site and reverse the sedation. Nalorphine was the first drug to be used as an opiate antagonist. The dose in equine is 8.8 μg/kg (0.40 mg/50 kg). Naloxone (narcan) is pure antagonist. It does not produce unpleasant effect. It is fairly short acting, therefore very large and frequent doses of naloxone appear to be necessary to counter the effect of the very potent, long acting analgesic, etorphine. The dose in equine is 9.9 μg/kg (0.45 mg/50 kg). Diprenorphine is a specific antagonist to etorphine and is very efficient in its role in animals.

Common non-narcotic analgesics:

Xylazine hydrochloride (Rompun): Xylazine hydrochloride is a potent non-narcotic, sedative, analgesic and muscle relaxant. It causes progressive depression of the central nervous system, leading initially to sedation, then at higher doses to hypnosis, unconsciousness and eventually general anaesthesia. The production of analgesia is dose-related and muscle relaxation is centrally-mediated. The muscle relaxant effect is a result of inhibition of itraneural transmission of impulse in the central nervous system. Bradycardia and transient cardiac dysrrhythmias occur when xylazine is given intravenously, however, these can be prevented by prior administration of atropine. The sedative effects are evident in 10 to 15 minutes after intramuscular injection and 3 to 5 minutes after intravenous injection and the sedation lasts for 1 to 2 hours and the analgesia lasts for 15 to 30 minutes. It is used successfully for control of colic pain in horses, and for conducting caesarean section and vaginal delivery in cattle. The dose in equines varies from 1.1 mg/kg intravenously or 2.2 mg/kg intramuscularly. The intravenous dose may be decreased to approximately 0.44 to 0.66mg/kg for most procedures as preanaesthetic medication. In bovines and caprines the dose varies from 0.055 to 0.11 mg/kg intravenously or 0.11 to 0.22 mg/kg intramuscularly. Twenty mg/ml solutions should be used to allow better control of the amount administered. Dosage in dogs and cats is 1.0 to 2.0 mg/kg intramusclurly or intravenously. Administration must be preceded by 0.04 mg/kg of atropine to avoid bradycardia.

15 Neurolept Analgesics

Central nervous system depression and analgesia produced without the use of barbiturate or volatile agents is referred to as neurolept analgesia. It involves the use of combination of analgesic drugs with that of tranquilizer/sedative. The combination of these agents is used for effectively alleviating the pain and they are valuable in facilitating restraint and handling of animals. The increasing practice of combination of analgesic agent with neurolept drugs (droperidol and phenothiazine tranquilizer) has expanded the number of preparations that the veterinarian can use for neurolept analgesia purpose.

The term neurolept analgesia is derived from two words, i.e., neurolepsia and analgesia. When the combination of droperidol (a neuroleptic or tranquilizing agent) and fentanyl (analgesic agent) as well as comparable agents were first administered in human beings to induce psychomotor sedation (neurolepsia) and analgesia, the genesis of this term evolved. Most opiod analgesics produce effect other than analgesia, and since most of these (e.g., nausea, vomiting, respiratory depression) are undesirable, a second agent is incorporated into the technique to counteract them. The so-called "neuroleptic" drugs used in this technique are tranquilizer which posses the ability to antagonize the emetic activity of morphine-like analgesics. Neuroleptic drugs reduce motor activity, decrease anxiety and produce a state of indifference. In dogs, this state produces analgesia and sedation to permit surgery, but muscle relaxation is poor and muscle movements may be elicited by auditory stimuli.

Acetylpromazine-Meperidine: This combination of equal volumes can be mixed and given for restraint. For small dose (7 to 16 kg) 0.5 ml is used while 1 ml is used for large animals.

Immobilon and other etorphine containing mixtures have been extensively used for the capture of wild game animals, e.g., elephants and giraffes which became sedated but remained standing. It is recommended for wild felidae (non domestic cats).

The effect of long-acting neurolept analgesia combination of drugs have been antagonized by opiate antagonist.

Composition of some commercially available neurolept analgesic mixtures.

Commercial name	Analgesic	Neuroleptic
Innovar Vet.	Fentanyl 0.4 mg/ml	Droperidol 20 mg/ml
Thalamonal	-do- 0.05mg/ml	-do- 2.5 mg/ml
Hypnorm	-do- 0.315 mg/ml	Fluanisone 10 mg/ml
Immobilon L.A.	Etarphine 2.45 mg/ml	Acepromazine 10 mg/ml
Immobilon S.A.	-do- 0.074 mg/ml	Methotrimeprazine 18mg/ml

Dissociative anaesthetics:

Ketamine: It is a powerful intravenous dissociative agent related chemically to phencyclidine. It has a shorter duration of action and its use has become more common in feline anaesthesia. In sufficient dosage, ketamine produced good analgesia. The characteristic "cataleptic" properties of this compound can be defined as a combination of little hypnotic potency and good analgesia. Hypertonous may often be present. However, higher doses associated with neuromuscular blocking drugs during the recovery phase by pre-treatment with benzodiazepines has substantially widened its spectrum of useful applications. Ketamine is unique among the intravenous agents in its cardiovascular stimulation that mimics increased activity of the sympathetic nervous system. The usual pattern of response follows a combination of vagal inhibition and adrenergic stimulation. The action of this compound is not clearly understood, but ketamine seems to interrupt cerebral association pathway while leaving the reticular activating and limbic system intact and depressing the thalamoneocortical system. The dissociative anaesthetic state associated with this drug is characterized by catalepsy, amnesia, profound somatic analgesia, near normal pharyngeal-laryngeal reflexes, and excessive skeletal muscle tone. Intramuscular injection of ketamine is usually painful, and restraint is advisable. Dosage range from 10 to 30 mg/kg, which will produce recumbency in 3 to 6 minutes and provide anaesthesia for 20 to 60 minutes. Acetyl promazine, 0.2 to 0.04 mg/kg intramuscularly, can be given with ketamine or, preferably, 10 to 15 minutes before ketamine injection. The mixture of diazepam and ketamine is a useful and effective combination. Equal volumes of these two drugs can be placed in the same syringe and given slowly at a dose of 1 ml/5 to 10 kg intramuscularly. It is also an excellent method for intravenous induction prior to maintenance with inhalation agents. Xylazine is commonly used with ketaminne in veterinary medicine. Ketamine is metabolized by the liver and also excreted unchanged by the kidneys. This drug should not be used in animals with hepatic and renal diseases.

16 Systemic and Toxic Effects of Local Analgesics

Local analgesics affect all types of excitable tissues including skeletal, smooth and cardiac muscle besides, nerve fibers. Their inadvertent delivery into systemic circulation results in side-effects, especially if the rate of absorption exceeds the rate of metabolism or elimination from the body.

The major target organs for the toxicity of local analgesics are the central nervous and the cardiovascular systems. Plasma concentration of a drug is mainly dependent upon absorption of the drug from the injection site, clearance of the drug from the blood stream to the tissue (tissue distribution), and elimination of the drug through metabolism and urinary excretion. Tissue areas with a good blood supply cause rapid absorption of the drug and rapid increase in plasma concentration similar to intravenous injection. Rapid absorption also occurs after application to the mucous membranes. Local analgesics of the amide type are largely bound to plasma proteins. Nevertheless, the concentration of the unbound drug determines the rate of disappearance of the drug from the blood stream and is also responsible for the biologic action of the drug and its passage across the placenta.

The local anaesthetic agent can produce both local and systemic toxic effects. Local tissue damage can be caused by solution of excessive concentration or by solutions in the wrong solvent, and by tissues undergoing necrosis. Systemic toxic effects follow the entrance of excessive solution into circulation, as for example following overdose, accidental intravenous injection, or too rapid absorption associated with rather slow breakdown. Toxicity is dependent on the type of the drug, rate of breakdown, concentration and speed of absorption, which is itself related to the vascularity of the particular part.

The amide-linked drugs are the most widely used local analgesics and have been subjected to extensive study. They are almost completely metabolized by the liver before excretion. Their metabolism is slower than that of the ester-linked agents. Hepatic blood flow is most important, and if liver perfusion is decreased as in congestive cardiac failure or if the liver is diseased (hepatic fasioliasis in cattle), plasma clearance concentration is decreased. The general condition of the patient also affects the toxicity of the anaesthetic drug; for example animals with liver damage have a slower rate of detoxification.

Local analgesics are removed from the blood stream by redistribution, metabolism and excretion. Highly perfused organs such as brain, heart, lungs and liver receive the initial bulk. Procaine and the related ester-linked anaesthetics are hydrolysed by esterases. Any interference with their metabolism by pathologic processes or drugs increases their systemic toxicity (e.g., heredity changes of plasma cholinesterase or decreased cholinesterase activity caused by pregnancy, liver disease or anticholinesterase drugs).

Toxic symptoms resulting from local analgesics are associated with cerebrum, and involve the nervous and circulatory systems. Central stimulation of nervous system causes excitement with giddiness and emesis. Convulsions are observed with higher doses. Death follows complete central paralysis from respiratory failure. In the circulatory symptom there may be centrally-induced hypertension and a small rapid pulse. Usually, however, peripheral vasodilatation is observed with a marked fall in blood pressure due to vasoconstrictor paralysis. In isolated cases of a sudden excess of local anaesthetic solution in the circulation there may be sudden heart failure caused by the block of nervous impulses in the cardiac musculature.

Treatment of toxicity: The treatment of toxicity caused by local anaesthetic solution is primarily symptomatic. By attempting to remove the effects of potentially fatal toxicity, life may be sustained until the natural destruction of the poison returns conditions to normal again. Signs of marked sympathetic stimulation (tachycardia, raised blood pressure, dilated pupils) may be controlled by sympatholytic drugs (phenothiazine derivatives), e.g., promazine hydrochloride at the dose rate of 0.5 to 1.0 mg/kg intravenously and a few drops of amyl nitrite on a swab to be inhaled.

With the development of convulsions small quantities of short-acting barbiturates (thiopentone, 5 mg/kg with intravenous diazepam, 0.1 mg/kg) are indicated to counter the cerebral stimulation. They should be given very slowly and in small quantities to the point when the spasm ceases, and afterwards repeated judiciously according to need.

The treatment should be prompt. Inhalation of pure oxygen is always very helpful. The use of nitrites helps in depressing blood pressure and reduces the tendency for convulsions to occur. In acute cardiac arrest there must be immediate cardiac massage as well as intravenous or intracardiac injection of 0.2 to 0.5 mg/kg adrenaline hydrochloride. Adrenaline stops the blockage of sensory stimulation to cardiac musculature. It is recommended that, after this intravenous injection of adrenaline, physiological saline or a similar solution should be given so that if there is circulatory arrest the drug nevertheless reaches the heart.

The central nervous system effects of toxicity are anxiety, restlessness, tremors proceeding to convulsions and respiratory failure. Toxicity usually follows over dosage, accidental intravenous injection, prematurely released tourniquet, or rapid absorption from vascular sites.

Recommended precautions while administering anaesthetic agents:

1. Use of minimal necessary doses of anaesthetic drug.
2. Use of minimal necessary concentration.
3. Aspiration should be done frequently to avoid venopuncture.
4. Use of vasoconstrictors into vascular areas.
5. Use of central nervous depressants prior to administration of local anaesthetic agents.

17 Acupuncture Anaesthesia

Acupuncture anaesthesia has been recently invented in China, where acupuncture anaesthesia is used as a useful working method for local or regional anaesthesia whereas, **acupuncture** is the most ancient form of therapy practised by Chinese for over 6000 years. The term '**acupuncture**' derived its name from Latin word "**Acus**" meaning needle and "**Punger**" meaning puncture. Acupuncture, in a literal sense is the art of insertion of needles into specific acupuncture points in the body, to relieve pain and to induce anaesthesia. The therapy by inserting a fine specially designed needle at specific points on the body is known as **acupuncture therapy**. These points are said to be linked in chains called **meridians** which in turn have internal connections to the organs. These **meridians** or **channels** run all along the body. It is believed that vital energy flows through these meridians. The specific points are known as acupuncture points which are small areas of skin about 1 to 3 mm in diameter. There are areas of skin with certain inherent qualities that set them apart from the rest of the body. They can be differentiated:

1. by their structure or histological picture,
2. by chemical sampling of tissues,
3. by their physiological behaviour, and
4. by their therapeutic role.

With the help of acupuncture point chart, the points are located within half an inch of the point. The electroacupuncture is used to exactly trace the suspect area. By criss-crossing the suspect area with the locator probe a point of maximum reading is obtained. This is taken as the acupuncture point. In order to stimulate a point effectively, some form of energy must be imparted to the point. Many forms of energy are currently used: mechanical, needling, thermal, chemical, light and electrical.

Electroacupuncture is the technique of applying current of various forms to the acupuncture points usually through needles.

It has very important role/application in acupuncture anaesthesia in animals. This technique was developed historically as an offshoot from manual manipulation methods already in use for various conditions. It is considered that electroacupuncture gives a stronger stimulation than plain needling, and it is more easily controlled, and is not tiring to the therapist. By using the acupuncture points, the anaesthesia can be produced by an electrostimulator within 20 minutes of induction period. With the help of machine (electroacupuncture), probe the exact location of the acupuncture points, insert the needle, connect an electrode to it, connect a return lead somewhere else on the body, turn the machine on, adjust the output to the maximum tolerable level, and leave it running for about 10 minutes. After a few minutes the patient becomes accustomed to that level of stimulation. Electric stimulation follows needle insertion. From lower setting, the frequency and voltage are steadily increased. The optimal frequency is about 30 to 50 Hz and the optimal voltage is the highest one tolerable to the animal. The degree of anaesthesia is tested by needle probes on the overlying skin. Surgery begins once there is no pain response. Since the electric current is being continuously applied, it is necessary to periodically adjust the voltage and vary the frequency as accommodation seems to take place with some loss of anaesthetic effect.

Acupuncture anaesthesia: The anaesthetic effects of acupuncture result from either electrical current of twisting action applied to strategically placed needles. These stimuli affect proprioceptors (the stretch and pressure receptors of the nervous system), thereby inducing a neurologic discharge that competes with and blocks out pain impulses coming from cutaneous nerves and other afferent pain receptors. Even pressure alone, without use of acupuncture needles, applied on certain proprioceptors has been known to induce surgical anaesthesia. This later phenomenon suggests that application of twitch on either ear or the muzzle of horse is a form of acupuncture-type anaesthesia. However, the acupuncture anaesthesia in China is employed successfully only in conjunction with barbiturates, sedatives, morphine, tranquilliser and local analgesia.

Acupuncture sites for regional surgery in equine: Yang Yan (San Yan Lo) consists of three acupuncture points, designated as San Yan Lo (FL_{23}), Yeh Yan (FL_{24}) and Chang Feng (FL_7). In the stimulation of the San Yan Lo points, local supplementary points are optional. On the other hand, in the stimulation of the ear points, they are mandatory. Supplementary local points are those near the site of the operation that are in the same dermatome. Anatomically, acupuncture needle insertion into FL_7 corresponds to needle insertion of or near the radial nerve. For San Yan Lo and Yeh Yan stimulation, the needle is inserted into San Yan Lo through the arm, to Yeh Yan. In this case the needle is inserted along median nerve. In general, anaesthesia is obtained by stimulating a nerve trunk anatomically related to the surgical area. The closer the needle is to the nerve trunk, the better the results. Best results can be obtained by stimulating the nerve trunk directly. Electroacupuncture is actually the stimulation of a nerve that ultimately affects the cerebral cortex. FL_{23} San Yan Lo (Three Yang Vein) is situated on the muscle groove, 2 cm below the tubercle of the radius along the lateral ligament of the fore arm. FL_{24} Yeh Yen (night eye) is situated on the medial side of the fore limb, near the cranial side of chest nut. FL_7 Chang Feng (wind chase) is present caudal and slightly ventral to the shoulder joint, in the depression between the long and lateral heads of triceps brachialis at the caudal margin of the deltoideus.

Induction of anaesthesia:

1. Two needles of the 4 and 6 inches respectively are used. The needle used for San Yan Lo and Yeh Yen is of 8 inches' length.
2. Apparatus: A semiconductor electric acupuncture machine.
3. Position of animal: The animal is left standing or in dorsal or lateral recumbency. The lateral position is preferred because, the needle insertion can be the same side as that of the operation. In a supine position, the needle can be inserted on the more convenient side.

4. Surgical operation: All three acupuncture points viz., FL_{23}, FL_{24} and FL_7 are used simultaneously for inducing anaesthesia required for different regional surgical operations in equines. For example, the operations in head region include enucleation of the eyeball, surgery for eye trauma and wound repair of the tongue. In neck region the operations are oesophagotomy, tracheotomy, laryngeal ventriculectomy and surgery for wind sucking and crib biting. The operations in thoracic region include thoracotomy, lobectomy and repair of pneumothorax. In abdominal region the operations are abdominal hernia, intestinal anastomosis, caesarian section and nephrectomy. And in pelvic region recanalisation of urethra, correction of vaginal hernia can be done. In addition orthopaedic surgery of limb can also be performed.

Ear acupuncture points for anaesthesia in equines (Fig. 37): The Chinese number 21 acupuncture needle is used. The depth of insertion is usually 10 to 15 mm. Insertion is bilateral.

1. Abdominal surgery: The heavenly gate, lung 1 (Fei 1) abdomen (FU) and triple burner (San chaiao) points are used.
2. Joint cavity: The heavenly gate and lung 1 points are used.
3. Fistula of parotid gland: The heavenly gate and lung 1 points are used.
4. Thoracic surgery: The heavenly gate, lung 1 and thoracic points are used.
5. Reduction of bone fractures in the limb: The heavenly gate occiput and kidney points are used.

The ear acupuncture points are supplemented by local acupuncture points in and around the site of operation. The needle is inserted in a slanting direction and is whirled during insertion. Electroacupuncture anaesthesia facilitates the successful completion of a range of operations in a fully conscious horse, mule, or donkey. Continuous electric stimulation is necessary to maintain sufficient excitation of central nervous system, so that reactions to pain caused by surgical trauma are continuously suppressed or abolished resulting in prolonged anaesthesia. The

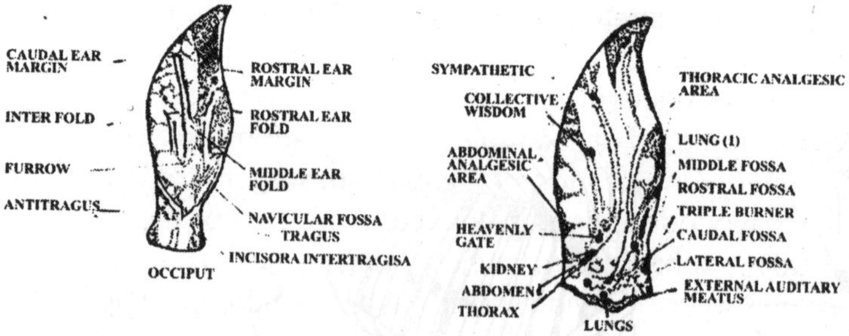

Fig. 37: Ear acupuncture points for anaesthesia in equines

observation that acupuncture is a satisfactory anaesthesia in equines has not gained popularity because of paucity of published clinical evidence (Hussain, 1995).

Acupuncture anaesthesia in cattle: The cows are restrained with nose lead. The acupuncture is performed and anaesthesia is produced only when the acupuncture needles are accurately placed in the acupuncture points. The acupuncture anaesthesia facilitated the performance of caesarean sections. The points used are Liver 14 and bladder 30.

BL 30 BAIHUHANSHU, is located at the caudal part of the lateral sacral crest and about 10 cm from the mid-dorsal line. The needle is passed subcutaneously downwards and forwards, to a distance of 1.0 to 1.5 cm. This point is bilateral.

Liv 14 CHIMEN, is on the lateral aspect of the thorax at the eighth intercostal space and in level with the shoulder joint. The needle at this point is passed subcutaneously to a depth of 3 to 4 cm in a downward direction.

Stimulation is achieved when the frequency is set at 180 to 240 cycles/minute (or 3 to 4 Hz). Voltage is increased until the skin begins to twitch. The stimulation is applied for 20 minutes before surgery begins. The site of surgery is the left paralumbar fossa (Fig. 38).

In dogs the needles are placed bilaterally in ST_{36} and GB_{34}, with electrical stimulation of an intensity such that localised tetany

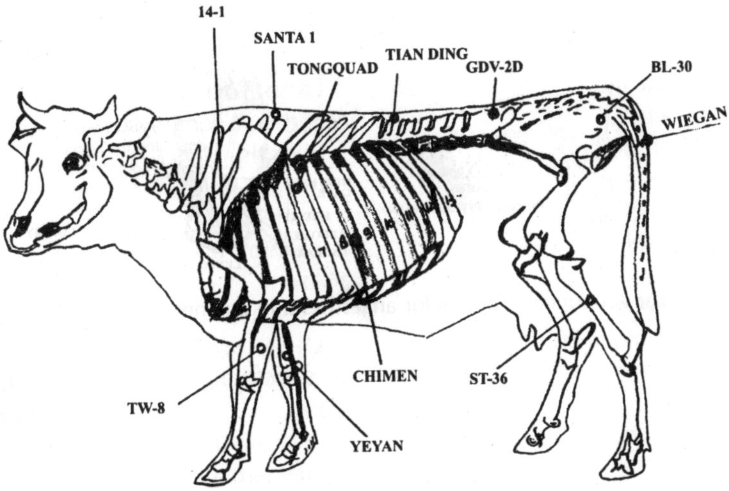

Fig. 38: Acupuncture anaesthesia in cattle

occurs. This will produce anaesthesia for surgical oophorectomy after an induction period of 20 minutes. Acupuncture anaesthesia in dogs is also produced by using the points Yan Vein (San Yan Lo) which consists of three acupuncture points, designated as San Yan Lo (FL_{23}), Yeh Yan (FL_{24}) and Chang Feng (FL_7). Their simultaneous stimulation enables the performance of surgical operations like hysterectomy, femoral head resection, perianal tumour resection, umbilical hernia repair and fracture repair with no adverse pain or other reactions

Index

Acepromazine 98
Acupuncture 3
Alcohol block 91-92
Anaesthesia 3
  Acupuncture 112-113
    In cattle 116-117
    In horse 114-116
  Therapeutic
    Technique of 34-49
  Local 16
    Action of 17-18
    Classification of 16-17
  Conduction 4
  Dissociation 4
Analgesia 3
  Continuous caudal 4
  Continuous spinal 4
  Electric 4
  Epidural 5
  Field block 5, 31
  Infiltration 30, 31
Intra-osseous 5
  Intravenous/regional 5
  Para vertebral 6
  Pressure 6
  Refrigeration 6
  Segmental 6
  Spinal analgesia 6
  Surface 5, 28
  Surgical 6
  Topical 6, 28
Anaesthesiologist 3
Anaesthetist 3
  Analeptic 3
  Anodyne 3
  Anaesthesiology 3
Anaesthetic 3
  Local, Toxic effects of 109
Autonomic nerve system 7, 96
  In cattle 69, 70
  In dog 72
  In sheep 72
Axolemma 3
  Axon 4
  Axoplasm 4
Basal narcosis 4
Benzodiazipine derivatives 99
Brain 8
Bupivacaine hydrochloride 26
Buprevnorphine 103
Carbocaine, see Mepivacaine
    hydrochloride
Catalepsy 4
Cataleptic 107
Chlopromazine 96
Cocaine 3
Combelen 98, 99
Dehorning 65
Diazepam 99, 100
  In cattle 100
  In goats 100
  In horse 100
  In sheep 100
Diprenorphine 104
Electropuncture 112, 113
Epidural analgesia 5, 83
  Anatomical consideration 86
  Complication
    Horse 87
  Lumbar 86
Etorphine 103
Fentanyl 102
Glycopyrrolate 95
Hyossine 95

Hypnosis 5
Ketamin 107, 108
Largactil, see Chlopromazine
Lidocaine 25
  In dog 25
  In horse 25
Lingual analgesia, see analgesia - local
Lorazepam 100
Marcaine, see Bupivacine hydrochloride
Meperidine hydrochloride 102
Mepivacaine hydrochloride 22
Methadone 102
Morphine 92, 102
Nalorphine 104
Naloxone, in horse 104
Narcosis 5
Nerve
  Pheripheral 10
  Spinal 12
Nerve block
  Auriculopalpebral 60
  Brachial plexus 77, 78
  Corneal 64
  Forelimb 69
  Hindlimb 79
    in dog 81
  Infraorbital 57
  Lingual 65
  Mandibular 66
  Maxillary 59
  Median 69
  Mental 68
  Paravertebral 50
  Peterson's 63
  Planter 70
  Pudic (internal pudeudal) 54
  Retrobulbar 62
  Saphenous 81
  Supra-orbital 58
  Tibial 81
  Ulnar 69
Neurolept analgesia 106, 107
Neuromuscular block 107
Opoid analgesics 101
Opthaine 25
Papaveretum 95
Parabiosis 36
Pentazocine 101
Phenothiazine derivates 95, 111
Procaine 24
  Blockade 37
Promazine 97
Rauwolfia derivatives 100
Ring block 32
Sedative 6
Sedative drugs 94
Spinal cord 7
Timgesic, see buprenorphine
Triflupromazine hydrochloride 97
Thiopentone 111
Thorazine, see chlorpromazine
Tranimul, see diazepam
Traquilizer drugs 94
Benzodiazepines 99
Valium, see diazepam
Xylazine 93, 104